DO IT YOURSELF

A Guide to Better Health

For You and Your Children

By Rabbi Dr. Yehonatan Sraya

A Holistic Approach

Name of book:
Do it Yourself - *A Guide to Better Health for You and Your Children*
By: Dr. Yehonatan Sraya C.A. Ph.D.
Translated: Yaffah Murciano
Jacket design, illustrations and general layout: Anna Khodorkovski
Published 2003 by the Israel Vegetarian and Vegan Movement
138 Allenby St., Tel Aviv 66522, Israel
Tel: 972-3-566-1975, 972-3-560-7774
Fax: 972-3-560-4582

Tele-fax: 972-2-643-5683
Tel: 972-2-642-4179
E-mail: DrSraya@hotmail.com

The information and suggestions in this book are not intended to replace the knowledge or abilities of a professional health practitioner. The sole purpose of this book is to provide a clear understanding of the holistic approach to various ailments and to serve as a self-help guide for overcoming them. The information contained herein does not apply to pregnant women, patients with heart problems, those recovering from surgery, or any other special condition. Always seek qualified health care when you need it.

Note:

Any diet specified in this book that does not tally with the principles of veganism and vegetarianism is recommended on a temporary basis only, for therapeutic purposes, in accordance with "It is time for the Lord to work, they have made void Your work," [Psalms 119, 126], and the principles set forth in the Rambam's *Mishneh Torah* and *Hanhagat ha'Beriut* (Healthy Practices).

Figures and footnotes are numbered separately in each section, and not continuously throughout the book.

In memory of Rolf, a naturalist, a poet, and a close friend
(1913–2001)

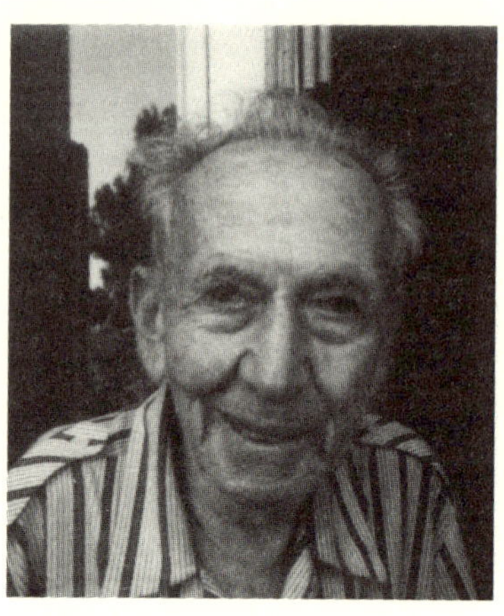

Changes

The book of life reveals another page
Your body changes slowly with your age
Just like your thoughts and mind, your needs and aims;
No longer are your hopes and tastes the same
Instead of passion, calm and patience came
When life was ready for a smaller frame
But softly, deep and darker burns your flame

Now with regret, you must watch your health
Success or failure seem to be not
Quite as important as they were before
So subtle are the changes that take place,
So different the problems that you face

Still, there are many blessings to embrace,
Life may yet be enjoyed in many ways

So full of beauty are the autumn days
Accept them humbly, with love and grace.

Rolf Redlauer
Jerusalem

Table of Contents

Acknowledgments:

First and foremost, I would like to thank my dear friend and esteemed advisor and mentor, Mr. **David Nachum**, chairman of the Vegetarian and Vegan Movement. May he continue his excellent work as director of the Movement for many years to come.

I am extremely grateful and extend special thanks to Mrs. **Chava Stroh**, secretary of the Vegetarian Society in Jerusalem. Her knowledgeable, helpful comments contributed greatly to this book.

Many thanks to Magister (Pharmacy) **Amnon Ozranski** who has advised me throughout the writing of this book.

My appreciation to my teachers,

Mr. **Ilan Horowitz**

Dr. **Moshe Olshevsky**

Dr. **Mina Ferne**

Dr. **Stephen Russell**, the "Barefoot Doctor."

Thanks to Dr. **Yom-Tov Hel-Or**, author of *Ripuy Vitali Tiv'i* (Vital Natural Healing).

Thanks to Professor **Yitzhak Levin,** founder of the Laboratory for Sleep and Dream Research at Bar Ilan University.

Thanks to my student, Mr. **Aryeh Krashinksi**.

My thanks to Mrs. **Sarah Tovah Wexler,** who edited a major part of this work.

My thanks to Mrs. **Varda Novick** for her devoted and dynamic editing.

My thanks to Mrs. **Yaffah Murciano** for her skillful translation.

My thanks toMrs. **Anna Khodorkovski** for her beautiful, accurate illustrations.

My thanks toMrs. **Chavie Frand** for proofreading and editing the final draft.

My thanks to Miss **Simone Rosenzweig** for proofreading the illustrated version..

Above all, I thank my loving wife, **Simcha**, who supported me throughout this project. Without her encouragement, this book would not have been possible. My thanks also to my wonderful children, who helped organize the material for this book.

Recommendations:

Do it Yourself - *A Guide to Better Health for You and Your Children*, by Rabbi Dr. Yehonatan Sraya, is what its name suggests: a guide to self-healing for people who have received standard, professional, medical treatment and wish to supplement their treatment with complementary medical practices.

Dr. Sraya, although not a Western doctor, has successfully combined elements of Western and Eastern medicine. This guide explains, in a clear and readable manner, the nature of various conditions or ailments, and provides treatment tips and guidelines that any person can follow.

The book also contains tips for healthy living and nutrition, according to the Jewish approach (the Rambam), the conventional Western approach, and the Chinese and Oriental approach.

The Guide provides those seeking to live a healthy life with tools for improving their health and understanding the nature of their illness.

I warmly recommend this book.

Professor R. Carasso, M.D. M.Sc.
Head of the Neurology Department
Hillel Yafe Medical Center, Tel Aviv

I became acquainted with Dr. Sraya at a course for practitioners, at which I taught a special method of Chinese acupuncture.

I'm very happy to know that he wrote a book, Do it Yourself - *A Guide to Better Health for You and Your Children,* in which he teaches people how to take care of themselves in the right way. This is a very meaningful work and I think highly of it.

It is definitely worth reading and applying Dr. Sraya's advice. Respectfully,

Professor Zhu Yu
Ganshu College of Traditional Chinese Medicine
Lenso, China

Dr. Sraya packs the book with charts and suggested resources. These, combined with the accessible, reassuring tone of his writing, makes this a very useful resource. I recommend it.

Dr. Roger Shaoul, M.D.
Certified Practitioner of Chinese Medicine (C.A.)
Lecturer, The Israel College of Naturopathy, Tel Aviv
(affiliated with the Israel Vegetarian Society)

Dr. Jonathan Sraya, an authority in many fields, has for many years dedicated himself to the practice of Chinese medicine. He is a regular contributor to our journal, *Teva-On ve-Beriut* (Natural Health), and has written many articles on healing, diet, herbal medicine, and healthy living.

This book deserves a place on everyone's bookshelf. It is a book to pass on to your children, relatives, colleagues, and friends. It is a book that will show you not only how to become healthy, but how to stay healthy.

David Nachum
Chairperson, The Israel Vegetarian and Vegan Movement

In this book, Dr. Yehonatan Sraya, a well-known specialist in Chinese medicine and related disciplines, describes common complaints, their causes, and how to treat them, in an attractive do-it-yourself program.

Even if you're not an advocate of natural or Chinese medicine, you will find this book an indispensable guide to understanding how we work.

Every home should have a copy of this book.

Shosh Navon, Naturopath
Chairperson, Naturology Department
The Israel Vegetarian and Vegan Movement

I am very happy to add my recommendation to Do it Yourself - *A Guide to Better Health for You and Your Children* by Rabbi Dr. Yehonatan Sraya. The author has dedicated himself for the past decade to intensive study of our Holy Torah and he received his Rabbinical Smicha from the Rabbinate of Israel at the Diaspora Yeshiva. Through his learning, Rabbi Dr. Yehonatan Sraya is uniquely qualified to write on the holistic approach to health, for the Torah Jew does not view the human body alone as forming a holistic whole, but the body and soul together form a holistic whole, and one who desires a healthy body must strive for a healthy soul as well.

Therefore, I warmly recommend his book and wish him blessings from Mount Zion and success in this and all his endeavors.

Rabbi Mordecai Goldstein
Dean and Rosh HaYeshiva
Diaspora Yeshiva Toras Yisroel
Mount Zion, Jerusalem

Introduction

Since a healthy and whole body manifest the way of the Lord, it is impossible to understand or know anything about the wisdom of the Creator if one is ill.
Rambam, Book of Knowledge, Chapter 4

These words of eternal wisdom make it vividly clear that, if we are to live according to our fullest potential, we must distance ourselves from anything that destroys our health and conduct ourselves in a wholesome and health-enhancing manner.

Good health is a blessing. To live joyfully, with good health, enjoying family and friends, is a blessing. In my work, I utilize techniques from both Eastern and Western medicine, to treat the *person,* not just the disease and help him acheive this blessing.

My goal in my practice, as well as in this book, is to combine and to make maximum use of both approaches. I firmly believe that both systems have valuable contributions to make towards reducing the suffering caused by a variety of symptoms and ailments.

As you will see, I place special emphasis on the techniques and perspectives of Eastern medicine because they take into consideration both the general cultural background, the personal constitution, and the specific complaints of the person involved. This is especially important, I believe, when someone is experiencing symptoms of anxiety or tension that can be connected with their personal situation and the reality of life in the 21st century.

Everyone can benefit and learn from the material included in this book. It was written especially for my patients, but it will also be useful for the general public, who can learn tools for self-help, including when to consult a professional practitioner. The information is general, yet specific enough to be of use to the layperson and the professional alike.

My hope is that you will be able to apply what you read here to help yourself, your family, and friends. My additional hope is that this work will lead you to look further into the various techniques and systems discussed here.

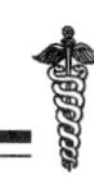

I. A Western Perspective

For the purposes of this work, I refer to Western medicine as the approach to health and wellbeing practiced by the "natural" schools of Western medicine. This definition includes techniques that until just a few years ago were still considered outside the range of "normal" healthcare.

In general, the standard Western, or "scientific," approach is to evaluate, diagnose, and treat illness "objectively." This approach relates to the symptoms of illness and what is determined to be the cause of the problem. However, in recent years, the Western medical establishment has become more open to healing approaches that are not necessarily of the scientific model, but which, never-the-less, produce documented results.

I discuss the following techniques because I find them to be very effective and use them in my practice. These descriptions are only meant to be an introduction to each subject. In practice, they are applied in a holistic and unique manner to each individual. I don't use all these techniques in any one treatment or with any one client. For self-help purposes, I suggest that you choose an approach that appeals to you.

Exercise

Whoever sits and does no exercise - even if he eats good food and takes care of himself according to medical practice - all his days he will suffer pain and his strength will be weakened.

Rambam, Book of Knowledge, Chapter 4

The negative effects of lack of movement on one's health were recognized thousands of years ago. This ancient knowledge has been proven repeatedly by medical experts in our generation, who tell us that exercise is vital to our wellbeing.

There is no greater blessing than physical vigor, and there is no bodily process that does not involve movement, often on a cellular level. No illness can be prevented or cured if the body's essential life-sustaining processes are not in order. Proper functioning is aided and enhanced by the effects of exercise.

The most desirable exercise is natural movement of the body, such as walking, running, swimming, climbing hills, and movement games. The most valuable exercise is that which speeds up the blood circulation, and therefore, the metabolism. Exercises that strengthen the spine and, in turn, have a beneficial effect on the nervous system are also important.

Exercise that can be done without excessive strain and that develops all parts of the body is the most useful. This kind of movement integrates the various systems and functions of the body and produces the most effective results. There are many kinds of exercise. However, what is more important than the type of exercise you choose is that you actually *do* the exercise, and do it *consistently*.

I personally feel that walking (and even speed walking) is the closest in pace to the natural movement of the body and, for this reason, is the most appropriate exercise for general strengthening and conditioning. Walking builds on the body's natural strengths and is the easiest to pursue consistently. No special equipment or location is required, only **commitment.** (Refer to Chapter VII - Exercise.)

Breathing

The quality of the internal chemical processes and exchanges that occur as a result of proper breathing is vitally important to your basic wellbeing. It is also important to realize that without breathing properly, it's impossible to achieve true relaxation.

Although this is not a detailed explanation, I can offer general suggestions for improved breathing. Any aerobic activity will increase your rate of respiration and thereby contribute to your general state of health. These include swimming, brisk walking, running, climbing stairs, sports, etc. The goal is to develop steady, rhythmic breathing that allows for a consistent and complete exchange of air.[1]

There are also a number of special breathing exercises that can be helpful in reaching this goal. The most useful are those that improve your rate of respiration and help to completely empty your lungs of the "old" air to make room for new, fresh air. The best way to do this is to exhale for longer than you inhale.

We can look at inhalation and exhalation as being representative of a "give and take" between our surroundings and ourselves. By improving our breathing techniques and abilities, we can improve our relationship with our environment.

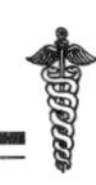

Autosuggestion

Suggestion means an influence which acts on the imagination and penetrates the subconscious. From the subconscious, this influence acts upon the autonomic nervous system to affect life and health processes, including those of relaxation.

Suggestion exerts itself through the conscious state of mind. The simplest and most direct method is autosuggestion, or self-suggestion. It is a method that is used commonly and is popularly referred to as "affirmations." For this practice to be most effective, it should be performed in a relaxed state, either lying on your back or sitting in a comfortable position. Then recite some chosen sentence(s) in a monotone. The best time to 'teach' yourself these sentences is before going to sleep.

For example: Every day my position improves in every way.[2]

Nutrition

Nutrition is one of the most important ways whereby you affect your general state of health. The food you ingest is what gives you the energy to function physically, emotionally, and spiritually. The importance of proper nutrition cannot be emphasized enough, especially in this age of fast foods. What the Rambam and the Chinese knew ages ago, we are now beginning to understand. You really are what you eat.

The modern Western diet is a relatively recent addition to the history of human nutrition. It is more an outcome of post-World War II advances in technology and transportation and the resulting financial special interests than a particular concern for complete nutrition. Much of what is taken for granted today in the West – particularly America – as a normal diet, is simply not healthy.

Just as we have begun to realize that smoking, pollution, and high levels of stress are not good for our health, we are also starting to realize that too much sugar, fat, oil, and animal proteins are also not healthy. There is no evidence to show that pesticides, preservatives, additives, and the assorted chemicals that are added to foods in the name of convenience are good for us at all. In fact, there are indications that the opposite is true – they may harm your health.

Western schools of natural medicine have a number of different theories when it comes to proper nutrition. It is advisable to learn about the theories and adopt one of them, according to your preferences. It is important, even if you are healthy, to consult with an expert to determine what kind of diet is best for your specific needs. If you are not well, that same expert can give you advice on ways to restore the body's natural balance through diet. (Refer to Chapter V - Nutrition.)

Be aware that drastic measures - such as fasting, enemas, or strict diets - without careful supervision - can cause irreversible damage.

Medicinal Herbs

The fruit thereof shall be for food, and the leaf thereof for healing. Ezekiel 47.12

Plants have been used for medicinal purposes since ancient times. We know that the prophet Samuel taught his disciples to use medicinal plants. From this perspective, the symptoms of illness are seen as the result of the body attempting to restore internal balance and harmony, and as far as possible, to limit the damage caused by the illness.

All treatment with medicinal herbs is directed towards strengthening the natural healing mechanisms that exist within the body and not merely treating the symptoms.

Medicinal plants are also used to create special preparations for feeding the nervous system and renewing its efficient functioning after a period of tension, or in cases of chronic weakness. This type of medicine is based on a holistic approach to health. It is aimed at assisting natural healing and restoring a balanced state of health to the patient.

The concept of illness, in this approach, finds its expression in the evaluation of the entire personality, the individual reaction to the illness, and the ability of bodily functions to restorate harmony and health.

Medicinal plants can be prepared in a variety of ways. In the past, herbs were mixed with food for their healing qualities as well as their pleasant flavor. Even today, many people make an infusion of herb teas or soak herbs for their useful qualities.

However, in a professional framework, those who practice healing with medicinal herbs tend to prescribe treatment in the form of tinctures. The practitioner can also prescribe solutions, gargles, ointments, and other preparations for external use. Pills, tablets, or capsules can also be prescribed.

The form in which the medicine is given depends both upon the problem and the plant itself. The practitioner needs to determine how the active ingredient of the plant will best be utilized, taking into consideration the patient's preferences and special circumstances.

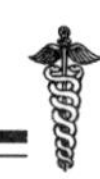

The potent combination of herbs and plants can affect the body in different ways. Pregnant women, especially in the first trimester of pregnancy, need to be particularly careful. For this reason, I recommend that you consult with an experienced practitioner. You are unique and only a qualified practitioner can tailor the medicine according to your special needs. (Refer to Chapter VI- List of Medicinal Herbs.)

Aromatherapy

Aromatherapy is the art of using the essences of aromatic oils that have been extracted from plants. Research carried out at various universities around the world report that there is clear evidence of influence on both the body and the mind from scented essential oils. Aromatic oils can aid a wide range of problems and are used for healing, pacifying the muscles of the body, releasing mental tension, and so on.

Aromatic or essential oils, like medicinal herbs, come from plants. The difference between the two lies in the parts of the plants that are utilized. Depending upon the family of plant, the oils can be found in the fruit, petals, flowers, the peel of the fruit, the plant's hairy gland, the channels, and the resin. Extracts of essential oils can be used in a number of ways, including taken internally, in the form of vapor, in a bath, in a compress, or massage. For proper treatment consult an experienced practitioner.

Reflexology

Every part of the body – every organ, limb, and gland – is reflected in the soles of the feet. Reflexes are actually found in all parts of the body, especially the hands, but the concentration of reflexes in the soles of the feet is particularly high, and is coordinated with the locations of the reflexive areas in the body. For example, the head is represented by the toes, the center of the body by the center of the foot, and the lower part of the body is represented by the heel of the foot (Figure 1 - Reflexology Chart).

Reflexology is based on the principle that if the body's limbs and organs are healthy, the soles of the feet will have no sensitive or painful spots unless there is an orthopedic problem. If a limb or organ of the body is ill or does not function properly, there will probably be sensitivity or pain in the corresponding location on the feet. The opposite is also true; if there is a reflex that is blocked, or degeneration in the soles of the feet for any reason (even from ill-fitting shoes), the corresponding limb or organ may feel the

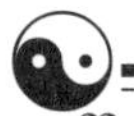

effects.

Pain and sensitivity on the soles of the feet are the result of a reflective reaction in the feet, in the to physical disease in the body's corresponding area.

A reflexologist massages the soles of the feet to stimulate the reflexes and improve blood flow to the entire body. Pressure on specific points causes the reflexes to "cleanse" blockages in the energy channels, by stimulating a specific bodily system – be it digestive, respiratory, etc. – to function to the best of its ability. Thus, the idea behind the treatment for constipation and diarrhea is the same; we are assisting the digestive system to become balanced and moderate, without extreme activity. As a result, the body relaxes and assumes routine, healthy functioning.

Very often, during treatment both therapist and patient feel a difference in the foot, as if there were "crystals" below the surface of the skin. It appears that there is an actual change in the tissue at these locations and that this change may be an indication of a problem in the corresponding organ or limb of the body.

If we lived radically different lifestyles, and walked or ran everywhere with our bare feet encountering various surfaces, we would naturally be healthier because of this continuous preventative "treatment." However, we lead relatively sedentary lives, spending most of our time sitting and wearing shoes that have been designed according to the latest style, rather than built according to the natural structure and function of our feet. Reflexology is the closest substitute for this "natural" massage. It aids and encourages the body to heal, using its own forces.

The advantages of reflexology are many, including:

☐ Simple, natural methodology
☐ Improve blood flow to the entire body
☐ Aid in cleansing the system, circulation, remove toxins and wastes
☐ Promote relaxation of tension in body and also affects the mind
☐ Precise diagnosis, through the soles of the feet

Before self-treatment, I suggest at least one session with a professional practitioner to obtain a diagnosis and instructions on where and how to press.

[1] Hel-Or, p. 83
[2] Hel-Or, pp. 163 -164

16

REFLEXOLOGY MAP

1. Head   (Pituitary, Cerebrum, Cerebellum)
2. Forehead, Brain
3. Cranial nerves
4. Temple
5. Eye
6. Sinus
7. Nose
8. Ear
9. Throat
11. Thyroid
12. Neck
13. Shoulder
14. Trapezius
15. Spine
16. Lung; Chest
17. Solar plexus
18. Heart
19. Adrenal Gland
20. Spleen
21. Small Intestine
22. Pancreas
23. Stomach
24. Duodenum
25. Liver
26. Gall Bladder
27. Ascending Colon
28. Transverse Colon
29. Descending Colon
30. Sigmoid Colon
31. Rectum
32. Kidney
33. Urinary Tract
34. Bladder
35. Sciatic
36. Ileocecal Valve

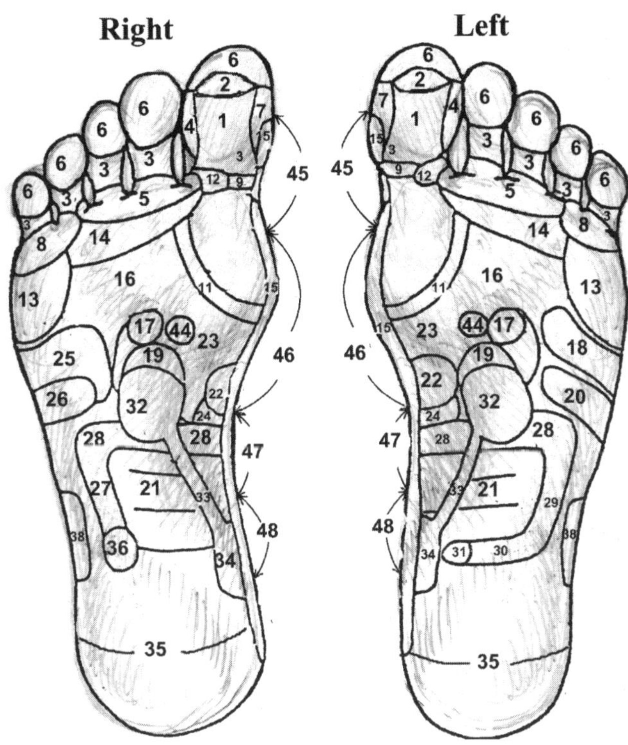

37. Knee; Lower Back
38. Uterine Tube; Spermatic Duct
39. Ovary; Testicle
40. Vagina; Penis
41. Uterus; Prostate
42. Groin
44. Thymus
45. Cervical nerves (7 c)
46. Dorsal Vertebrae
47. Lumbar Vertebrae
48. Sacral Vertebrae

Foot (Side)

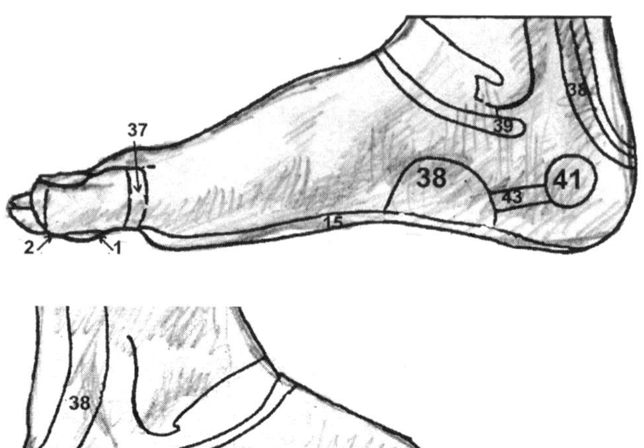

Foot (Top)

1.   Head
2.   Forehead, Brain
6.   Sinus
10. Tonsils
13. Shoulder
14. Trapezius
15. Spine
16. Lung; Chest
37. Jaws
38. Knee; Lower Back
40. Ovary; Testicle
41. Vagina; Penis
42. Uterus; Prostate

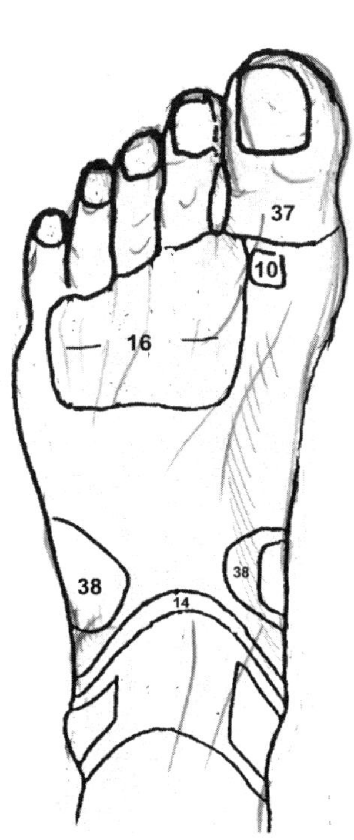

 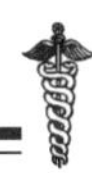

II. An Eastern Perspective

In order to understand what I refer to as the Eastern approach, we must first become aware of a few concepts. Although this system is often referred to as Chinese or Oriental medicine, it is a misnomer to call it "medicine," since, in fact, it embraces a whole world outlook. It deals with an entire way of life including diet, physical exercise, breathing techniques, and meditation as well as other aspects of lifestyle.

Eastern medicine, which is really a school of thought or philosophy, encompasses the whole person, viewing the patient as a unique entity and taking into consideration his family background, culture, community, and environment. The Eastern approach to health problems places less emphasis on finding the cause of the problem and, instead, looks for the lack of balance that is produced as a result of the problem.

Indeed, in Oriental cultures, the healer was traditionally not considered a doctor, according to our way of thinking. The healer's role was that of teacher, educator, guide, or advisor. Responsible for looking after the health of patients and preventing illness, the healer was not paid when a patient fell sick. Having failed to foresee what would happen and supply proper guidance to fortify the patient as needed, the healer would be compelled to reorganize the patient's way of life, taking into account eating and sleeping habits, as well as exposure to fresh air and sunshine. Proper guidance related to diet and healing herbs, as well as appropriate exercise and relaxation techniques would be provided. And if this didn't help, various healing techniques were utilized.

The following are some basic concepts of Eastern (Chinese) medicine, which differ from the Western perspective. They include:

- Energy
- Yin/Yang
- Function of the Organs
- Five Element Theory
- Meridian Theory

Energy

Energy (*chi,* in Chinese) has many functions, and according to the Chinese way of thinking, is comprised of both substance and force. The substance is derived from our parents – through genetics – and from the nourishment we obtain from the food we eat and the air we breathe. This substance of *chi* is found in the organs and the meridians that flow through a person's body and is connected with the blood, the nerves, and beyond, as "some sort of electricity." The force of the *chi* – connected with movement – is what propels the substance through the meridians to the limbs and the tissues, enabling them to function properly. Eastern medicine aims to both preserve and balance the *chi* within the body.

Yang/Yin: Male and Female He Created Them Genesis,1:27

The Lord G-d formed man from the dust of the earth (yin). *He blew into his nostrils the breath of life* (yang).

Taoist's (from the Chinese word *dao,* meaning 'way') believe that harmony – between man and the world, between man and himself, between the polarizing forces of the universe and in each detail of it – is essential to leading a healthy, productive life. They group the elements of the universe into forces of *yin* or *yang*. These forces can dominate one another and even destroy each other. However, without both *yin* and *yang*, man cannot exist.[1]

Everything in the world can be attributed, either wholly or partially, to the forces of *yin* and *yang*. Like most concepts in Eastern medicine, these qualities do not actually exist in a material fashion but are concepts, or influences, which impact on our physical reality.

Yang, to a large extent, represents the masculine aspect and is characterized by activity, heat, speed, aggressiveness, and striving for cold. *Yin* generally represents the feminine aspect and is characterized by passivity, introverted behavior, quietness, and striving for heat. However, it is important to remember that the definitions of *yin* and *yang* are not absolute. Everything is relative and a wise person recognizes that any given situation is never black and white. For example: A tree trunk is *yin* relative to a stone, but a stone is *yin* relative to metal. Likewise, water is *yin*, but hot water is more *yang* than cold water.

Like everything else in the universe, the organs are also classified as either *yin* or *yang*. The *yin* organs are relatively solid and important internal activity occurs within them. They include the heart, lungs, liver, spleen,

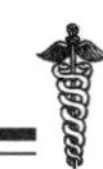

and kidneys. The *yang* organs are hollow and transference activity takes place within them. The *yang* organs include the small intestine, large intestine, gall bladder, stomach, and bladder.

Yin Organ(solid, internal)	Yang Organ (hollow, transference)
Heart	Small intestine
Lungs	Large intestine
Liver	Gall bladder
Spleen	Stomach
Kidneys	Bladder

Yin/Yang Organ Table

Function of the Organs

There is some similarity in the way Western and Eastern medicine perceive the physiology of the human body. Both agree, for example, that certain organs are responsible for the pumping and circulation of blood, others for the digestion and assimilation of food, and yet others for the absorption and storage of fluids. However, there are also many differences between the two systems, arising mainly from the fact that Chinese medical theory, when it first evolved, steered clear of operations, as far as possible. Therefore, in Chinese medicine, the anatomical model is based on the external appearance of the organ.[2]

I shall describe the functions of the various organs in pairs (*yin* and *yang*), as is standard practice in Chinese medicine: Lungs and colon, spleen and stomach, heart and small intestines, kidneys and bladder, and liver and gall bladder.

1a. *The lungs*: The lungs control breathing. The lungs draw the air in and down and, with the help of the kidneys, distribute it to the various organs of the body. Psychologically speaking, the lungs represent "give and take." Pathological symptoms may be excessive perspiration, or asthma, which is a psychosomatic phenomenon.

1b. ***The colon***: The colon is responsible for eliminating waste matter. Psychologically speaking, the colon represents "letting go." People who find it hard to let go (retentive personalities) tend to develop constipation.

2a. ***The spleen***: The spleen controls the digestive process, the absorption of fluids and solids, and also the breakdown of food and its conversion into energy. Psychologically speaking, the spleen is linked to the brain, and represents the ability to "coordinate and organize."

2b. ***The stomach***: The stomach is important for the initial breakdown of food in the body and for a general feeling of wellbeing.

3a. ***The heart:*** The heart is responsible for circulation of the blood. Psychologically speaking, it accommodates the spirit, and is the source of the feeling of joy. Pathological states may find expression in depression, sleep disturbances, etc.

3b. ***The small intestine***: The small intestine separates digested food from undigested food. Psychopathology: When a person becomes "incensed," small blood vessels burst from the "heat" and blood is secreted in the urine.

4a. ***The kidneys***: The kidneys, as the seat of energy, are second, if not first, in importance in the hierarchy of organs. They mix a person's innate energy with the energy derived from air and food to convert it into the body's basic energy (in Western medicine, the adrenal gland). Psychologically speaking, the kidneys are responsible for the "fight or flight" response to situations of fear and danger. The kidneys are also responsible for fluids and blood production.

4b. ***The bladder***: The bladder stores urine prior to its voluntary secretion. Situations of tension and anxiety may give rise to an involuntary secretion of urine and bedwetting in children.

5a. ***The liver***: The liver cleanses and purifies the blood. It is responsible for the free passage of blood through the body. Psychologically speaking, the liver controls feelings of anger and frustration. Tension causes the blood to stop flowing, resulting in a feeling of frustration, or heats the blood, causing it to rise to the head, resulting in feelings of anger ("it makes my blood boil").

5b. ***The gall bladder***: The gall bladder stores the bile prior to its secretion. It is closely linked to the liver. Psychologically speaking, the gall bladder governs the tendency toward melancholy, anger, or fear.

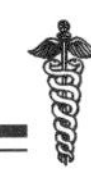

Five Element Theory/Organ Correspondence

A later school of thought introduced the concept that the world is made up of elements. According to the Greeks, as well as the Rambam, there were four elements. The Chinese, however, introduced a fifth element. The five elements are fire, earth, metal, water, and wood. Each element has corresponding organs.

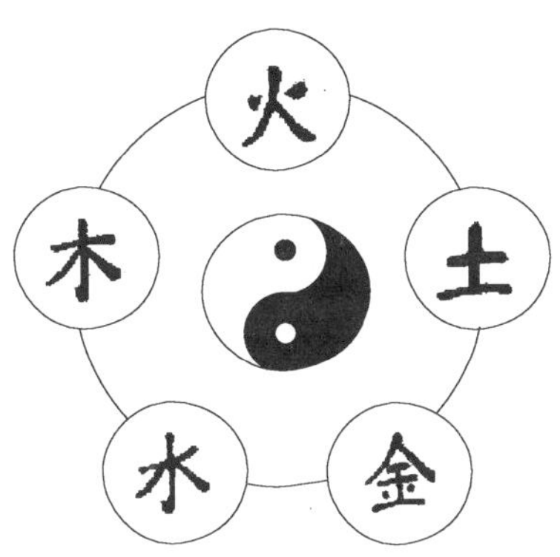

Over time, a fusion occurred between the theories of *yin* and *yang* and the five elements. In line with this fusion, the *yin* organs were paired with *yang* organs. Each pair of organs corresponds to the element of the *yin* organ. Each element also has a color that characterizes it, and a part of the face to which it corresponds or "opens," as do the organs. In addition, each element has a particular part of the body that it "feeds," and an emotion that characterizes it. The following table clearly illustrates all the correspondences.

It is interesting to note that the Chinese do not make reference to a healthy soul in a healthy body. Instead, each organ is seen as having an emotional or psychological function (part of the soul), to which it gives expression.

	Fire	**Earth**	**Metal**	**Water**	**Wood**
Organ	Heart/small intestine	Spleen/ stomach	Lungs/large intestine	Kidneys/ bladder	Liver/gall bladder
Opening	Tongue	Mouth, lips	Nose	Ears	Eyes
Body Part	Face	Eyelids	Skin	Bones	Nails
Tissue	Blood vessels	Muscles	Body hair	Hair on head	Ligaments/ tendons
Color	Red	Yellow	White	Blue/black	Green
Emotion	Joy, laughter	Sadness, introversion	Sorrow, nostalgia	Fear, groaning	Anger, shouting

Five Element/Organ Correspondence Table

Meridian Theory

According to Chinese medicine, there are meridians, or channels, in the body that run beneath the surface of the skin and between the muscles. Each meridian has its own specific location, path, and direction through which the energy flows. There are twelve major meridians in the body. Ten of the twelve meridians correspond to an internal organ and are referred to by the name of that organ (Figures 1 - 10 Meridian Channels).

Along the length of each meridian are numerous points that can be used to achieve therapeutic goals. In order to maintain physical and mental health, the meridian pathways must remain open, allowing the *chi* to circulate freely. A blockage or obstruction along the course of a meridian causes impaired circulation of the *chi* and can lead to disease, which in turn leads to further blockage of the meridian. Blockages can be due to physical or mental (emotional/spiritual) causes. Opening the meridians and keeping them open can be achieved in various ways. The best known and commonly used techniques are acupressure, acupuncture, and massage.

The meridians are also classified as *yin* or *yang,* depending upon the organs to which they correspond. In general, the *yin* (or female) organs are more internal and the *yang* (or male) organs are more external. The flow of *chi* in the *yin* meridians moves from lower to upper, and the direction of energy flow in the *yang* meridians is from above moving downwards. The meridians are divided into those of the hand or the foot, which indicates where the energy channel begins or ends (Figures 11 and 12 - Meridian Channels, see page 33).

In addition to the twelve primary meridians, there are also secondary meridians that do not directly correspond to any internal organ. The most important of these secondary meridians are:

- Governing Vessel, which governs all the *yang* meridians as well as the flow of energy in the back part of the body in addition to other functions of the body (Figure 13, see page 34).

- Conception Vessel, which governs all the *yin* meridians, seemingly bisects the front part of the body and is associated with conception and genetic functions (Figure 14, see page 34).

Figures 1-14 can be found at the end of the chapter.

Following are Eastern techniques for working to restore and maintain a balanced state of health:

24

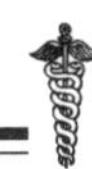

- Movement and Meditation

- Shiatsu, Acupuncture/Acupressure

Movement and Meditation

Modern medicine is beginning to acknowledge the close connection between mental state and illness, a concept that was recognized by sages of previous times and has been passed down through the generations in the form of various traditions. A number of Eastern cultures have movement and meditation systems that were created, and have continued to evolve, to help balance the mental and physical energies in the human body for improved and enhanced health. Two of these systems are Tai Chi and Yoga.

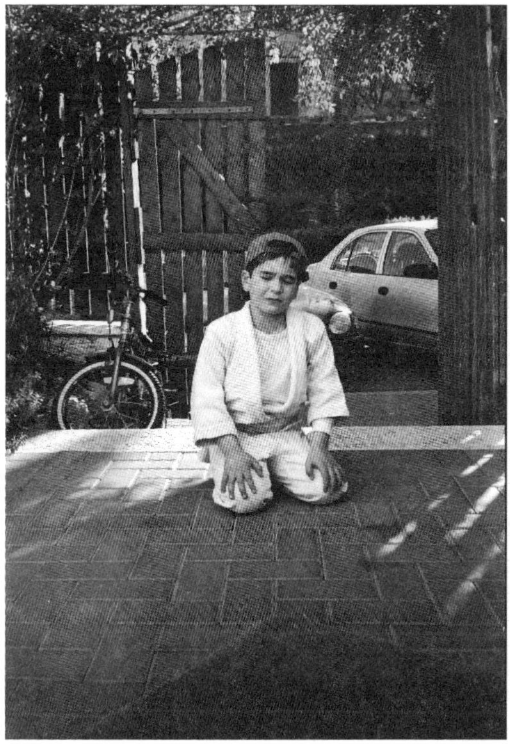

Tai Chi

Tai Chi is an ancient Chinese martial art that has evolved into a form of exercise aptly called meditation in movement. When practiced regularly, Tai Chi brings about a state of balance between all five elements and between the *yin* and the *yang* in the body, as well as between the body and the universe at large. As a result of this "energetic" state of balance, mental relaxation and tranquility are experienced.

The feeling of communion engendered by the practice of Tai Chi can provide a proper perspective from which to view emotions. This leads to tranquility and lack of tension, which in turn increases self-esteem and therefore makes a valuable contribution to general wellbeing.

The physical aspects of Tai Chi enhance overall fitness by improving equilibrium, flexibility, and dexterity. Movement becomes more efficient and energy is used more productively. Recent research has shown that Tai Chi, when practiced regularly, can markedly decrease physical frailty, particularly in the elderly.

I recommend the practice of Tai Chi as an entire form, not just one or two exercises. The combination of meditation and movement can have profound spiritual as well as physical effects. The choice of time and place for practicing Tai Chi are of great importance – no distractions and an ample supply of fresh air are vital.

Yoga

Yoga is an ancient Indian system. Its goal is to raise the body and mind above their limits, to improve one's state of existence. Yoga has a physical component as well as a highly developed spiritual component – meditation.

If the physical aspects of yoga are practiced carefully and persistently, a person's thoughts will become calm and emotions will become less volatile. At a higher level, control can also be developed over bodily sensations, allowing the individual to neutralize the connection between pain or stress and disease.

Combining the meditative practices, in which the intellect controls the thoughts and emotions, with the physical positions and breathing exercises of yoga can bring about an indescribable balance of mind – especially under stress. This tranquility enables the true self or soul to operate without any distortion. This is totally different from the state of tranquility brought about by drugs.

Shiatsu

The word "shiatsu" is comprised of two Japanese words, meaning "finger" and "pressure." Combined, these words express the main principal of this simple, yet effective, system of treatment. By exerting finger pressure on specific points, shiatsu treatment releases blockages and opens the meridians for uninterrupted energy flow. Because the meridians correspond to the

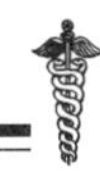

organs of the body, balance among the various organs of the body is also achieved. Shiatsu works to preserve or restore the body to a state of balance as well as to activate the mechanism of self-healing. After a shiatsu treatment, the patient feels more at ease, balanced, and relaxed. The body works more smoothly and the patient feels regenerated and refreshed.

Originating in ancient China, this Japanese method of treatment is intended to relieve pain and tension while inducing relaxation, enhanced energy, and a feeling of wellbeing. The choice of points and meridians for treatment is the result of wisdom developed over thousands of years in China, and of continued methodical development for scores of years in Japan. Shiatsu is often referred to as acupressure, which is based on a form of acupuncture. One of the great advantages of shiatsu is that you can do it yourself.

How shiatsu works is not entirely understood, but it does work. A few of the possible explanations are:

- Pressure on key points activates a specific substance in the brain, which causes pain relief in general and in certain organs in particular.

- Pressure exerted on key areas of the body disperses surplus lactic acid that has built up in muscle tissue and can cause various problems and diseases.

- Pressure on certain points produces electrical-like stimulation, which causes blockages in the energy pathways to open so that the natural balance and activity of the organs can be restored.

Shiatsu is closely related to acupuncture and works according to the same principles. It activates essential channels of energy – the meridians. However, instead of using needles, as in acupuncture, shiatsu uses finger pressure to exert influence upon the meridians and their energy.

Unlike reflexology, which exerts energy indirectly and in a general way on certain organs, shiatsu treats the organ or meridian in need of activation directly. This is accomplished by working on very specific points (either local or distal) that are specifically connected to the organ while reflexology works on zones.

Shiatsu differs from Chinese massage in that pressure is exerted on specific points along the meridians with dry fingers rather than with the aid of oil, as in Chinese massage. In either case, the aim is the same: to restore balance and harmony.

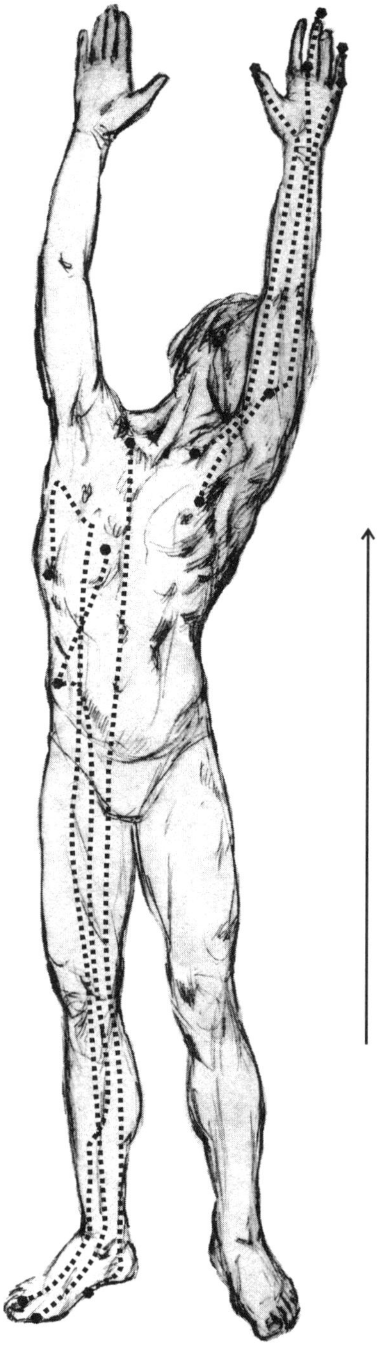

Yin Meridians
Figure 1

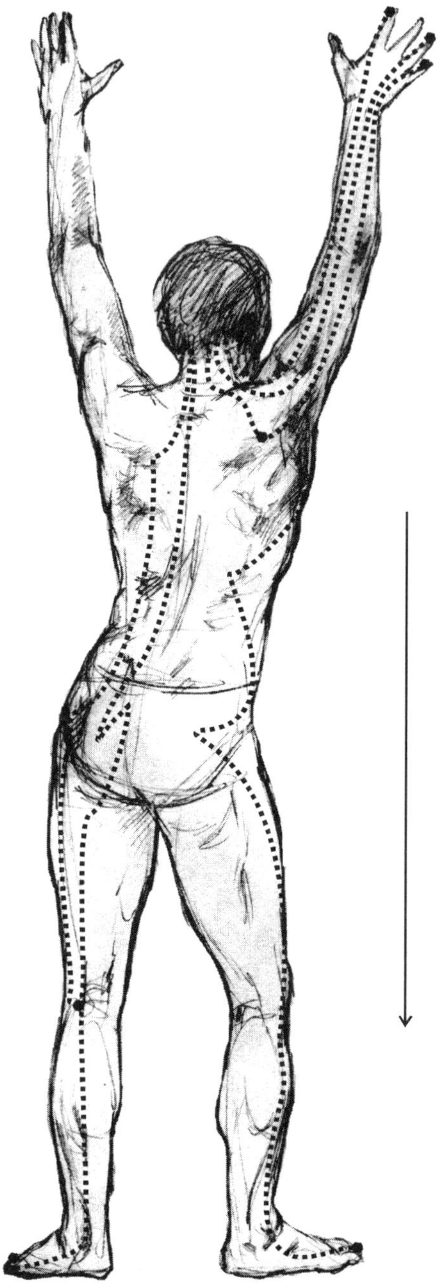

Yang Meridians
Figure 2

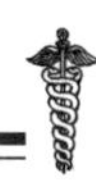

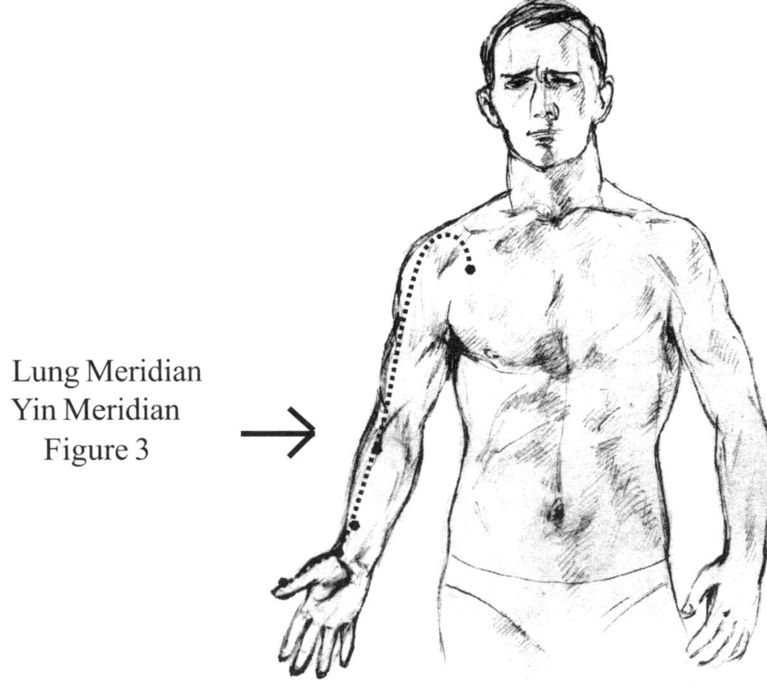

Lung Meridian
Yin Meridian
Figure 3

→

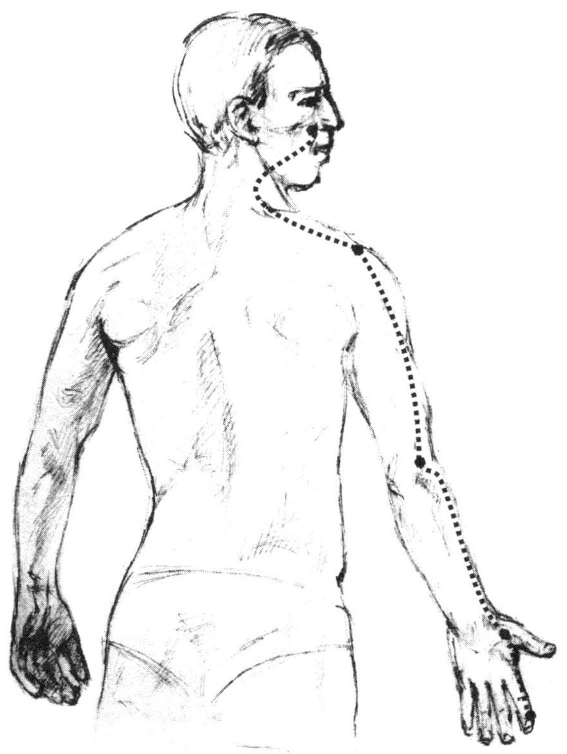

Large Intenstine Meridian
Yang Meridian
Figure 4

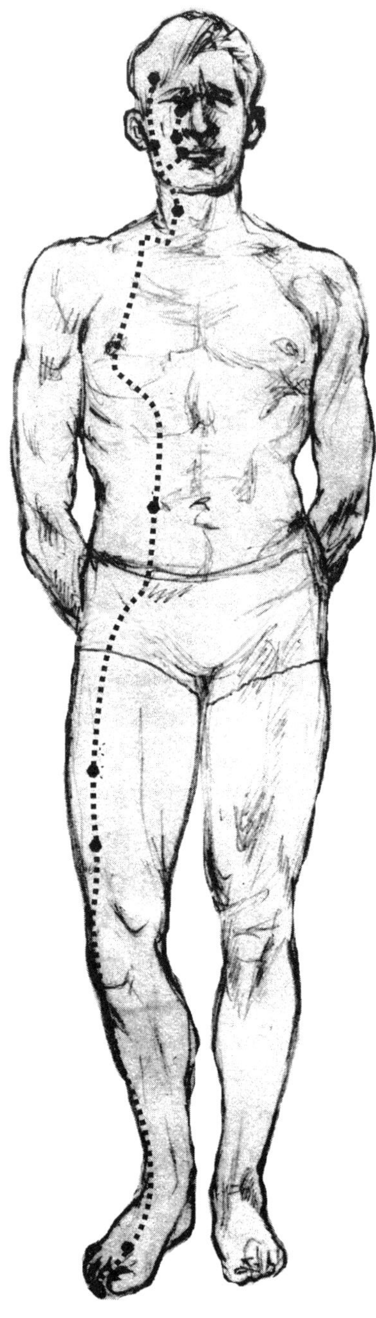

Stomach Meridian
Yang Meridian
Figure 5

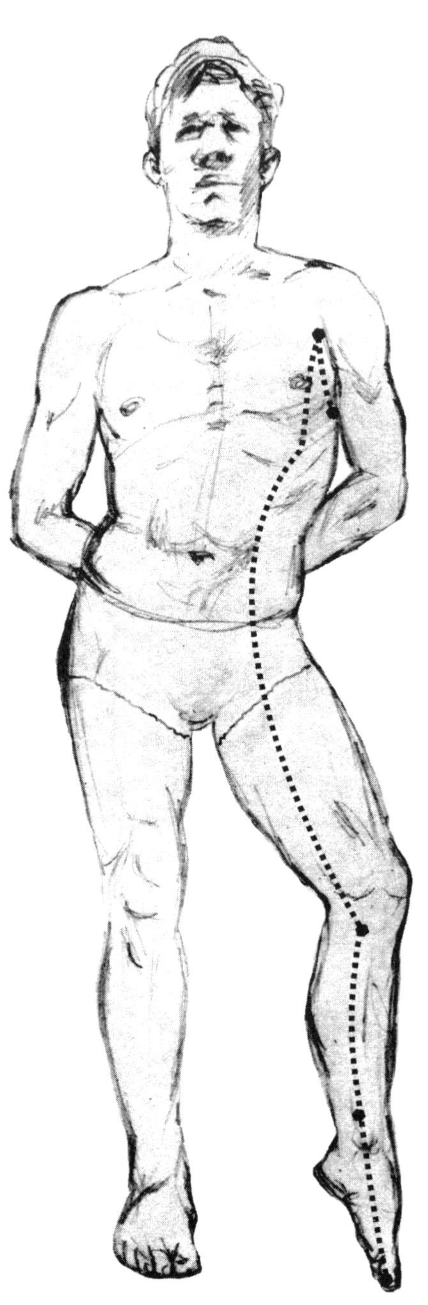

Spleen Meridian
Yin Meridian
Figure 6

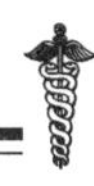

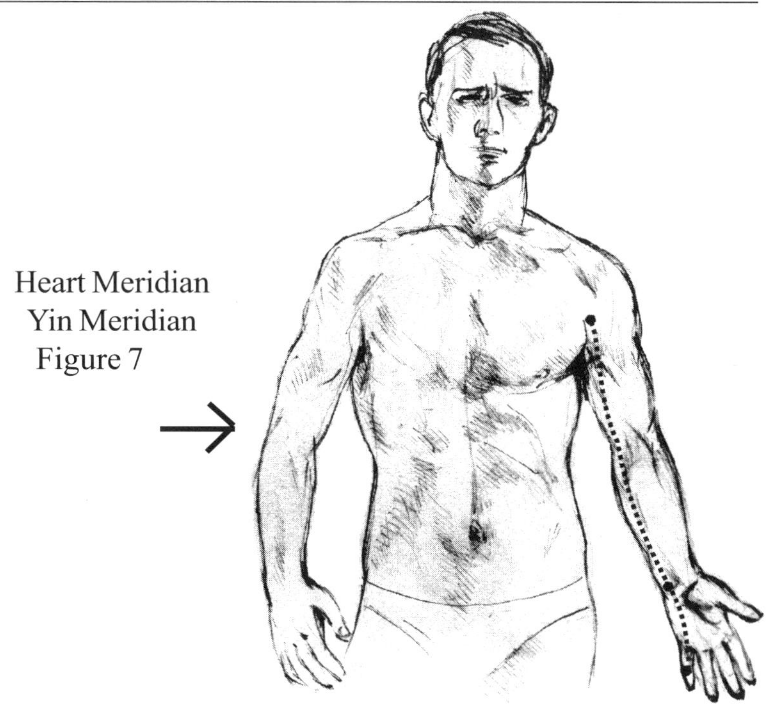

Heart Meridian
Yin Meridian
Figure 7

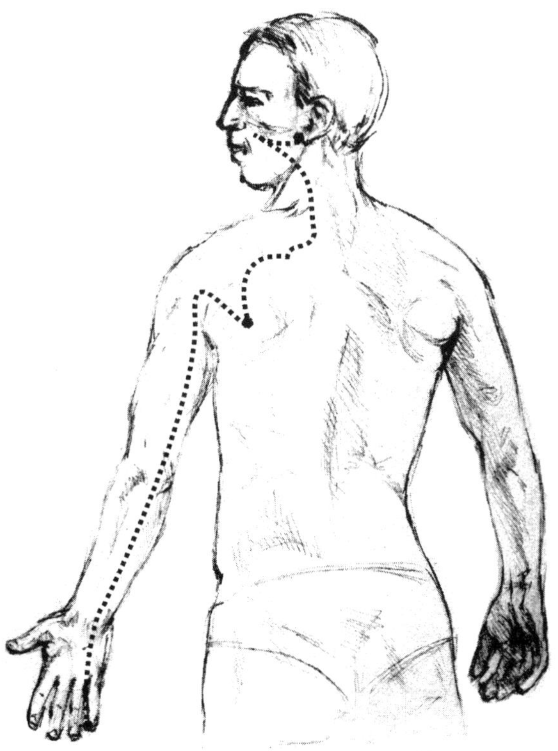

Small Intestine Meridian
Yang Meridian
Figure 8

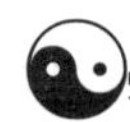

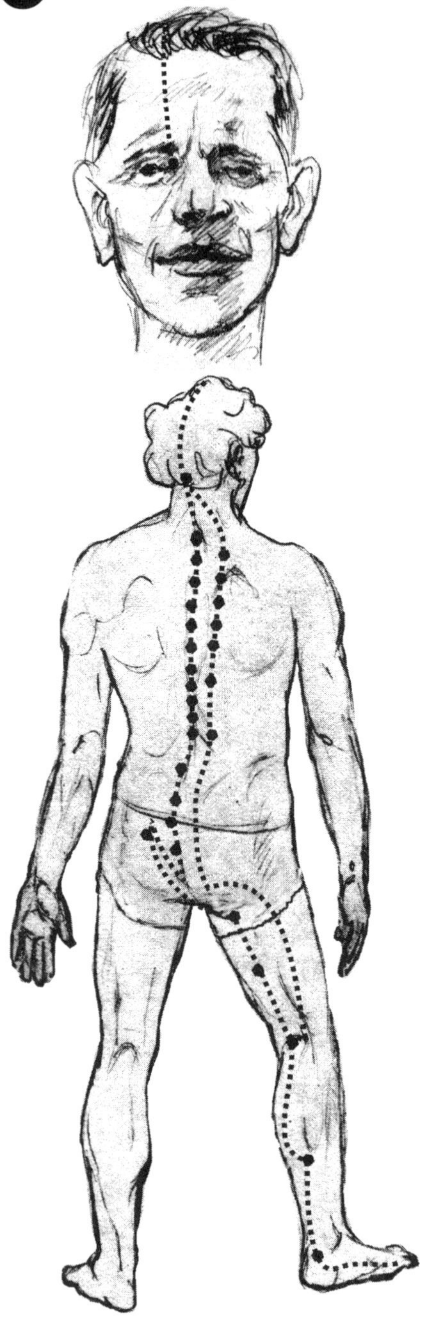

Bladder Meridian
Yang Meridian
Figure 9

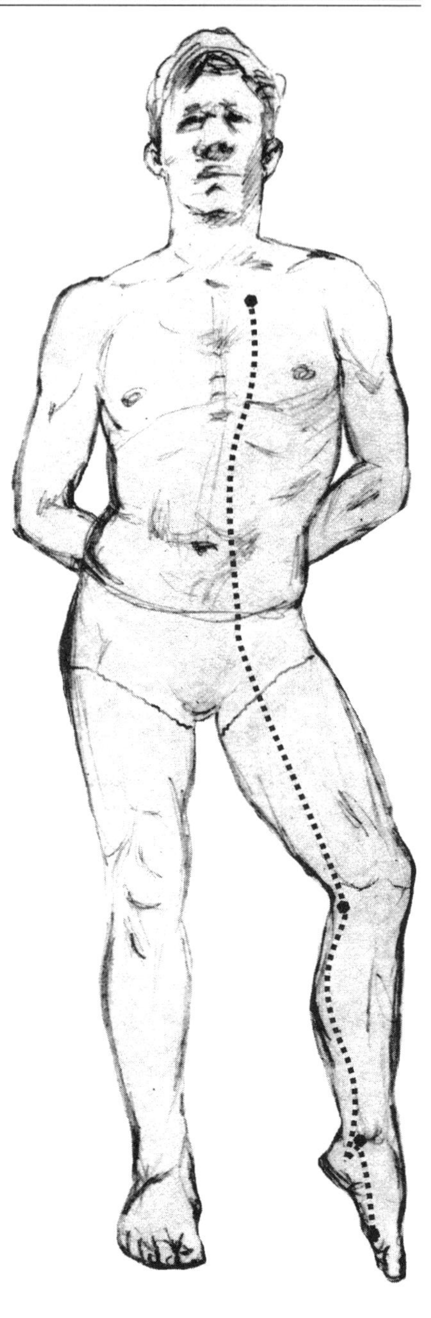

Kidney Meridian
Yin Meridian
Figure 10

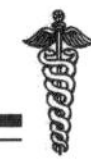

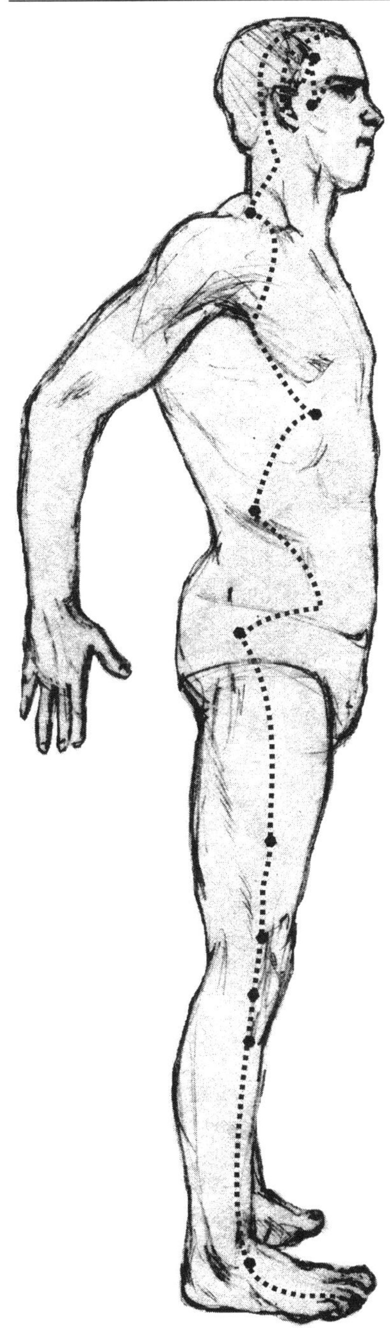

Gall Bladder Meridian
Yang Meridian
Figure 11

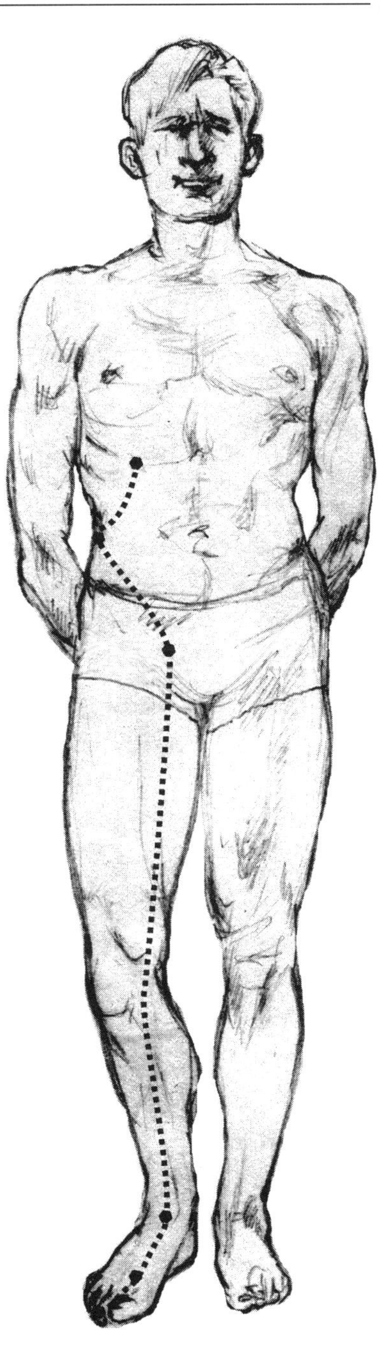

Liver Meridian
Yin Meridian
Figure 12

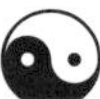

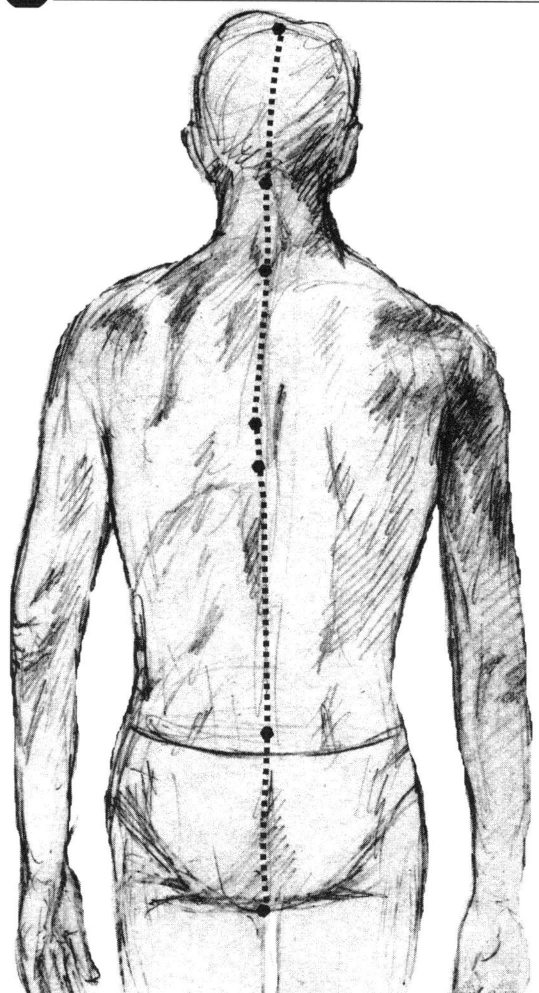

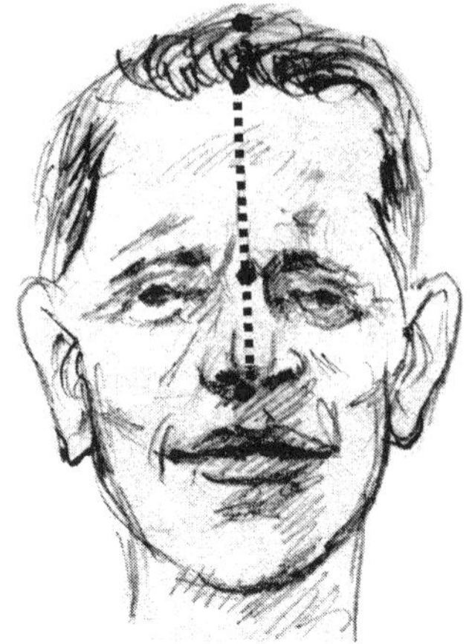

Governing Vessel
Figure 13

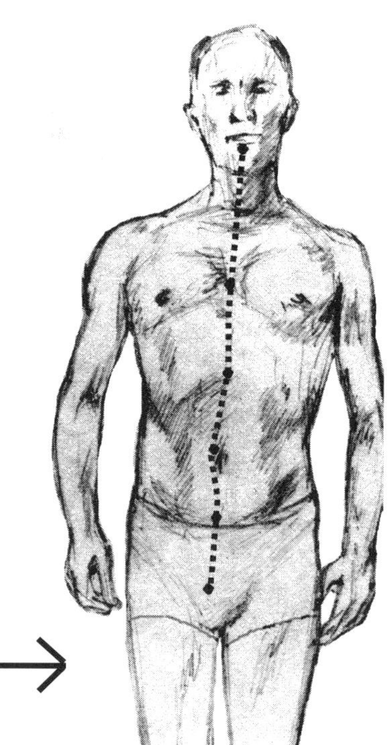

Conception Vessel →
Figure 14

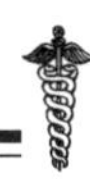

III. Various Ailments

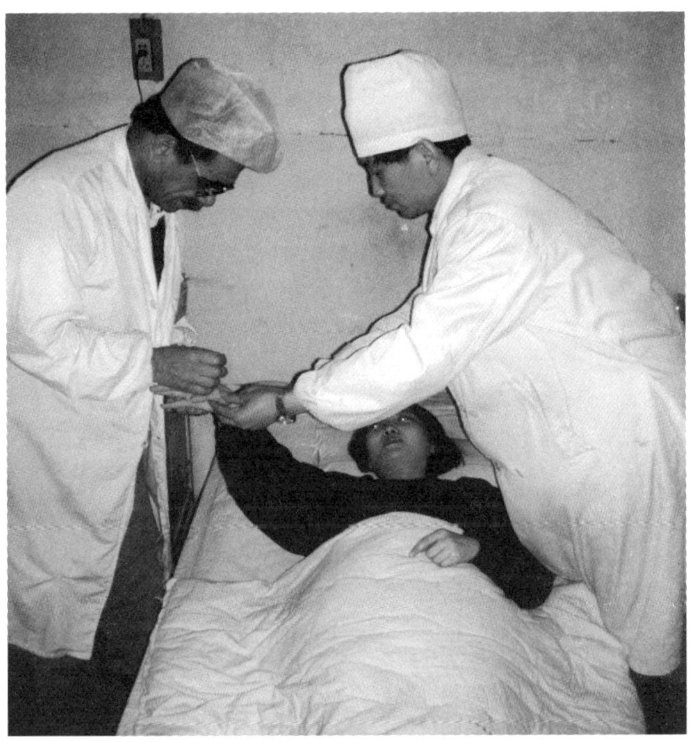

Please note:

1. After familiarizing yourselves with the causes of the ailment, carefully read Chapters One and Two, paying special attention to the reflexology chart and the map of meridians before proceeding to the treatment stage.

2. The numbers in the reflexology chart refer to zones.

3. The numbers in the shiatsu and acupuncture figures refer to specific points. Measurements that are cited in fingerbreadths are based on the breadth of the patient's finger, not the healer's (in the case of children, this can represent a significant difference).

4. Any reference to vitamins in this book relates to food supplements that contain these vitamins. Naturally, vitamin capsules provide vitamins in more concentrated form, but the food containing the vitamins is more balanced and has supplements that cancel out the side effects that accompany the ingestion of pure vitamins.

5. In shiatsu and acupressure, press on **both** sides of the body.

Allergies

Allergies are one of the common health problems confronting Western civilization. Whether it is seasonal hay fever, food allergies, or environmental allergies, this problem is affecting an ever-increasing number of people. Adults and children are equally affected and, depending upon the intensity of the symptoms, can suffer from mild to severe distress.

An allergy is an over-sensitivity to a specific substance or substances. The symptoms of allergy can be extremely varied and may include: sneezing, runny and/or itchy nose, rashes, shortness of breath, swollen face, tearing eyes, migraines, diarrhea, flatulence, vomiting, and constipation. Because the symptoms can be so varied, and are similar to those of other health problems, allergies are often overlooked as the cause of the suffering. This can cause the problem to become chronic, and the allergic reaction is repeated over and over.

During an allergy attack, the body perceives a threat from certain substances, whether or not any danger actually exists. The immune system responds to this perceived threat immediately and manufactures antigens to respond to the "dangerous" substances. (These "dangerous" substances cause no reaction in people who are not allergic.) The antigens "attack" the substance, causing a physical reaction – the allergic reaction.

One way to describe an allergic reaction is with the following scenario. Imagine an emergency state of high alert, with a nation-wide call up of defense forces, air-raid sirens blaring and defensive missiles flying through the air. Everyone leaps into action, only to later discover that it was a false alarm. An overexcited intelligence unit mistook a passing herd of sheep or goats for a hostile army – a simple case of mistaken identity.

In the case of an allergy, the intelligence unit does not learn from its past mistakes, but simply repeats them over and over. Each time, the entire warning and preparation system is set in motion with the same degree of intensity as before. As you can see, a commission of inquiry would be useless here.

In other words, the immune system causes the body to go into a state of alert, setting off a powerful chain reaction, each time a certain substance is perceived as harmful. What triggers this response in some people and not in others is the million-dollar question.

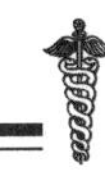

The most common allergens – substances that cause allergic responses – are pollen, foods, and animals. Dust and environmental or chemical substances, such as laundry detergent, can also cause allergic reactions in susceptible people. Although any food can cause an allergic reaction, certain foods seem to be more common offenders. These include milk and dairy products, chocolate, eggs, wheat, oats, rye, and various grains, due to the blend of proteins they contain. Some people have an allergic reaction to soft drinks, perhaps because of the additives and preservatives they contain. Sometimes a certain combination of foods may produce a reaction. Some people also have an allergic response to certain medications or antibiotics.

Although allergies are not fatal, they can make life very difficult. One of my patients came to me after suffering for years from migraine headaches every Sunday. In the course of treatment we discovered that he was having an allergic response to the fish and *hammin* he was eating on *Shabbat* (The Sabbath). Another of my patients spent his nights in the early spring in an armchair because his allergic asthma was seriously aggravated at that time of year. Sometimes people will have an allergic reaction to foods that are not common to their culture or geographic part of the world.

It can be extremely difficult to isolate the cause of an allergic response. There are people who suffer from allergic reactions without even knowing they have an allergy. Others know they have an allergy but don't know what causes it. Sometimes the allergen can be narrowed down to a category such as a medication, animal, or plant, but it's not clear exactly which type of medication, animal, or plant is causing the reaction.

The most difficult allergies to isolate are food allergies. There are various techniques used by doctors and healers to detect the cause of an allergy. One possibility is to eliminate any suspect foods from the diet and replace them with other foods. This is a complicated process, however. Another method is to eliminate all food, except for whole-grain rice, and then gradually start introducing other foods into the diet, one at a time. This is also an involved technique and requires you to record every single food you eat, space the addition of new foods, and check your pulse rate after each meal.

It is very difficult to prevent allergies because usually there is a genetic tendency towards an allergic response (though it is sometimes latent), and because it is almost impossible to avoid contact with allergens. The best defense is to strengthen the body's natural immune and defense systems. A strong and balanced body is less likely to have intense allergic responses.

There are a number of steps you can take to help yourself deal with allergies including diet, herbs, relaxation, acupressure, and massage. I have outlined some general suggestions below.

Diet

♦ Eat natural, fresh, and whole-grain foods, without added preservatives and additives, as much as possible.

♦ Include plenty of calcium-rich foods in your diet such as sesame seeds, tehina, and dark-green vegetables.

♦ Use garlic. It is not only a natural antihistamine, but also a natural antibiotic. Garlic is especially effective when combined with propolis, and can be taken in capsule or tincture form as well as eaten raw. Parsley will eliminate the offensive odor associated with garlic.

♦ Eat foods rich in vitamins. Vitamins, particularly vitamin C, can strengthen the immune system. I strongly recommend professional consultation before taking vitamin supplements.

Reflexology

♦ Give a general massage, especially to the big toe and upper sole.

♦ Press # 1,2,3,4,5,6,7,16, and 44 (Figure A).

Herbs and Supplements

The most effective herbs are:

♦ Echinacea (Cone Flower), which strengthens the immune system.

♦ Equisetum (Horsetail), which is an anti-allergen.

♦ Siberian Ginseng, which serves as a tonic, specifically for the adrenal

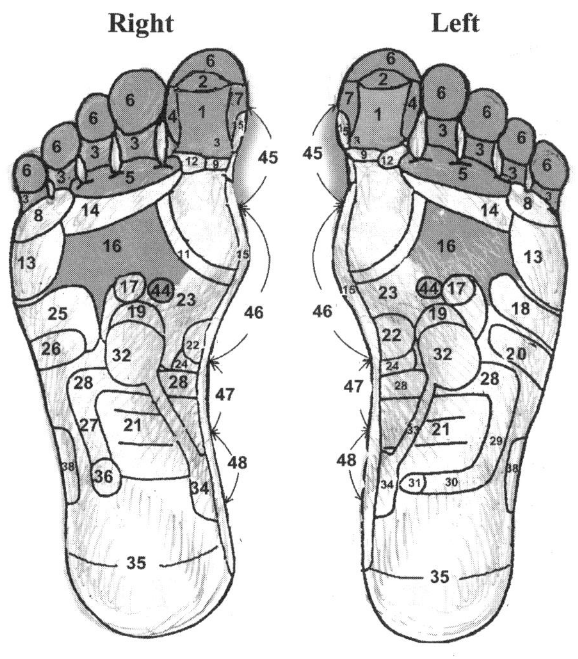

Figure A

38

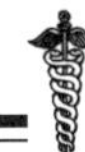

system and the body in general.

♦ Propolis, which contains general restorative properties.

Relaxation

Stress and tension weaken the body's immune system, rendering a person more sensitive to external stimuli, including allergens. Almost any relaxation technique as well as regular exercise, such as rhythmic breathing and swimming, can be very helpful in reducing negative physical responses to stress. Yoga is particularly effective.

Acupressure, Shiatsu, and Massage

According to Chinese medicine, allergies are the result of a weakening of the body or loss of energy in the body, particularly the lungs. The main focus of treatment should be on strengthening the body in general and the lungs in particular.

☐ Blocked or runny nose

Press on the following points:

♦ Adjacent to the nostrils on either side of your nose (see Figure 1,a).

♦ Middle of your upper lip (see Figure 1,b).

♦ Between the eyebrows (see Figure 1,c).

☐Lungs Acupressure

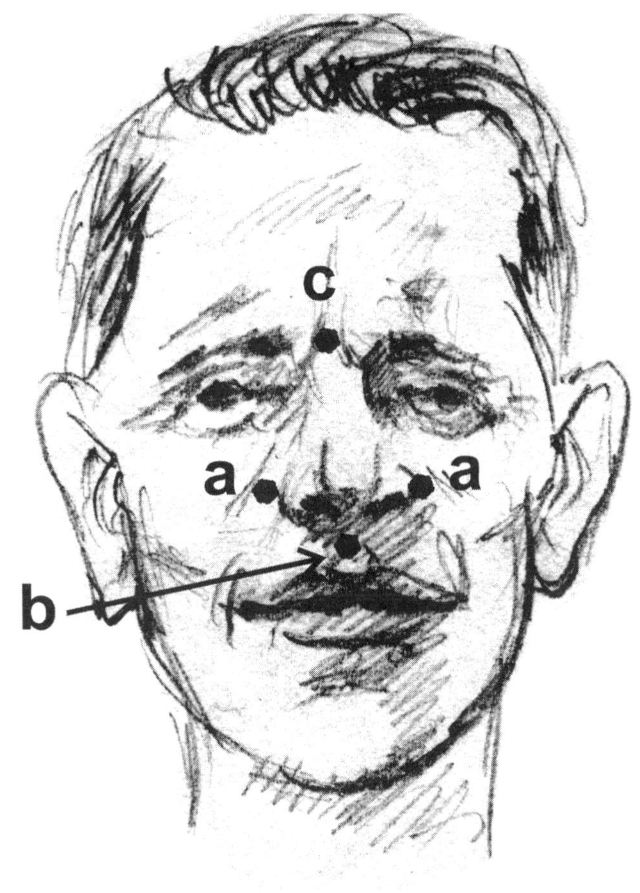

Figure 1

(acupuncture without needles) and massage should be applied to the muscles between your ribs, on your chest, and to the corresponding area on your back between your shoulders.

❑ Sore Throat and General Aches and Pains

◆ Press the point located where your thumb and index finger meet. Use the opposite thumb and press as hard as you can tolerate in the direction of the inner bone (on the palm of your hand) (Figure 2).

❑ Cough and Breathing Difficulties

◆ The point near your wrist that lies about two inches away from the fleshy part of the thumb (Figure 3).

◆ The point is on the inside of your elbow, near the biceps (upper arm), level with the thumb when your elbow is partially bent and your palm is facing up (Figure 4).

❑ General Strengthening

◆ The point is located in the soft tissue of the lower leg about four fingerbreadths below the kneecap, one fingerbreadth from the outer edge of the shinbone (Figure 5).

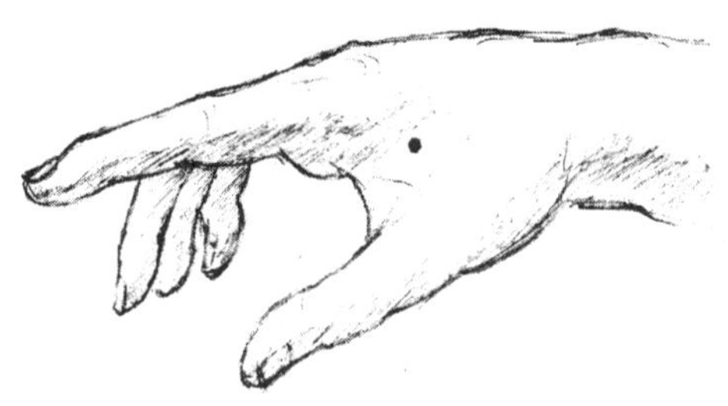

Figure 2

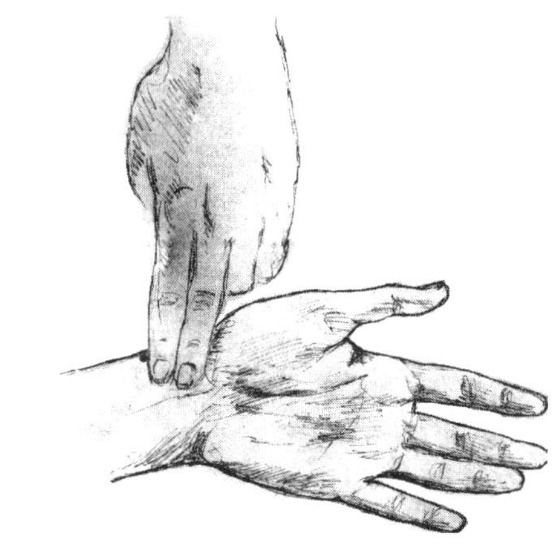

Figure 3

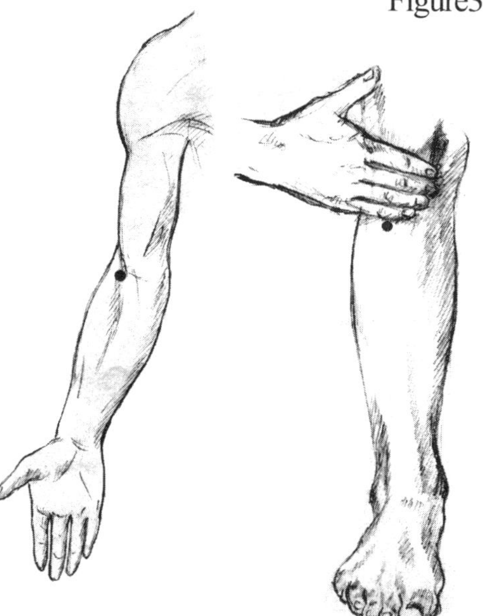

Figure 4   Figure 5

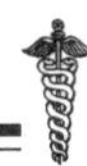

Back to Basics

In 1982, during the Lebanese War, I spent days and nights cramped in a narrow, cold armored vehicle. After a while, I began to suffer from neck and lower back pains. I had to move around gingerly, and it was only after walking, movement, and exercise that my muscles began to relax.

When I returned to civilian life, my doctor told me to stop walking from Bayit Vegan to the Kotel,(Western Wall), as I occasionally did. My orthopedist also told me off for practicing karate. "At your age," he said, "You shouldn't be doing karate." The result of all this advice was that I went around doubled over with pain.

I subjected myself to various treatments, including physiotherapy, but all to no avail. One of the more extreme treatments I had was mechanical neck traction. Unfortunately, the machine was apparently not properly adjusted, and instead of pulling my neck, it pulled my jaw out of shape. As a result, I walked around for a month with a distorted face. (I was not yet familiar with alternative practitioners.)

Luckily, a shiatsu practitioner came to the rescue. With acupressure and exercises, I slowly returned to myself, and resumed my walks to the Kotel. I did not, however, go back to karate, which is a pity.

Was my neck problem solved? Although the underlying problem remained, I no longer suffered from neck and shoulder pains, or the attendant headaches. Did my lower back problem disappear? To a large extent, the pressure on the disc disappeared, although the area was still sore. I felt that even a small straw could "break the camel's back."

Nowadays, in order to keep healthy, or when my neck starts "seizing up'"or I feel the beginnings of pain, I do acupressure and exercises. All in all, I try to prevent a flare-up by daily acupressure, daily tailor-made exercises, and weekly participation in a Yoga and Feldenkrais group.

What caused the neck and back pains?

The neck and lower back pain were symptoms of two different phenomena:

The neck - There were (and doubtless still are) age-related degenerative changes and diet-related arthritic changes. The pains were due to an acute attack, which "exploited" a chronic susceptibility. There was friction between discs in the neck, which caused the pain. The body, wishing to defend itself, sent a message to the muscles via the central nervous system ordering them to contract in order to protect the exposed and painful nerves. However, the muscles continued contracting long after it was really necessary.

Lower backache - The backache had a different cause. It was the result of a shift in the normal pressure that is usually exerted on the discs between the vertebrae. When pressure was exerted on one side of the disc, the disc moved slightly sideways, pressing on nerves passing from the back to the buttocks and feet. Once again, as with my neck problem, the pain activated the body's defense mechanism, causing the neural muscles to contract. The problem probably resulted from a clumsy movement due to the uncomfortable position I was in or from lifting a piece of equipment the wrong way. No doubt the neck problem also affected my back. Although the cause of the pain was different, the result was almost identical. In both cases, the local muscles were stiff.

These two problems are fairly representative of most types of neck and back pains. The tremendous confusion regarding the types and causes of backache makes it difficult for us to explain the phenomenon. Some doctors offer explanations that are difficult for the patient to understand. Some of the more common terms used by doctors are: arthritic changes of the spine, spondylitis, scoliosis, kyphosis, lordosis, trauma, sciatica, or muscular contraction.

I shall attempt to explain each of these terms.

1. *Arthritic changes* result from inflammation of the joints. It can be systemic, i.e., involving the whole body, or can affect specific joints only. Once it spreads to the spine, the situation is chronic and hard to treat.

2. *Spondylitis* is an inflammation of the vertebrae in the back. In a chronic inflammation, a person will feel stiff after lying down or sitting for a while. The stiffness eases after walking, movement, or other physical activity.

3. *Scoliosis* is curvature of the spine. This usually occurs during adolescence, when the adolescent suddenly "shoots up," or at middle age.

4. *Lordosis and kyphosis* are both distortions of the spine's natural "S" shape, in which the person's back either becomes humped or flat. These can be caused by any of the above conditions, or by lack of exercise, causing a weakening of the stomach and back muscles. Bad posture, incorrect sitting position, a paunch, overweight, and pregnancy may also cause these conditions.

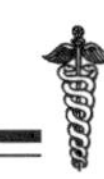

5. ***Trauma, slipped disc, or lumbago*** cause acute or chronic pain, sometimes with painful spasms or cramps. The attacks erupt from time to time, because a series of tendons, discs, or even muscles have been stretched, subjected to excessive pressure, or have "clenched."

6. ***Sciatica*** – inflammation of the sciatic nerve occurs when the thigh nerves are over-stimulated due to pressure on a disc in the lower back area. The resultant pain radiates out along the hip and thigh, and down to the foot. When there is an acute attack, the pain can become unbearable. The patient cannot fall asleep, and cannot even lie comfortably, except perhaps in one position that he discovers through "trial and error."

7. ***Muscular contractions*** *(back or neck cramps)* usually result from the aforementioned problems. Cramps are the body's defense mechanism to protect sensitive nerves. The body continues to defend itself long after it is really necessary. A stiff neck can also result from a draft or from sleeping under an open window.

8. Finally, there is a ***psychological component*** to many neck and back pains. The expression "stiff-necked" is synonymous with stubbornness and obstinacy. Many people who are angry or tense suffer from a stiff neck or backache.

There are also more serious problems such as a ruptured or fractured disc, osteoporosis, bone diseases such as gout, or tumors.

Treatment

a. ***Rest or exercise?***

For the first few days, when the pain is particularly acute and it is hard to move, sit, or even lie down, you're best off lying down. Once you are in this position, you may try doing gentle movements. Do not lie on your stomach, since this intensifies the pressure on the discs and nerves. The best position is on your back with your knees resting on cushions, in order to take the pressure off the lower back. In more serious cases, lie on a carpet and rest your feet on the seat of a chair – forming an angle of 90 degrees between legs and thighs, and between thighs and back.

If you prefer lying on your side, place a thin cushion between your knees, to remove pressure from the discs and nerves in the lower back.

For those who prefer lying on their stomach, do so only after the more acute stage is over. Lie in a semi-fetal position, on the side of your stomach, with one leg bent.

b. *Heat or cold?*

This is also a very individual matter. For some people, a cold compress on the vertebrae of the lower back or neck helps. Others prefer a hot water bottle or electric cushion. However, **general** experience shows that in the acute stage, a cold compress is more helpful, while in the later stages when the patient is on the mend, or in chronic cases, heat is more helpful.

c. *Should you wash the painful area or keep it dry?*

Some people find that a hot shower helps. A strong jet of water that gets hotter and hotter until the heat is almost unbearable is effective. If you like baths, be careful when getting in and out of the tub. A salt bath can help relieve muscle cramps. Take a packet of coarse salt, empty it into the bathtub, fill the bathtub with boiling water until it is a quarter full, and then add cold water until the heat is bearable. Soak in the bath for about 20 minutes to half an hour. Rinse the salt off in clear water, without soap. Afterwards, lie down for half an hour.

d. *Massage with/without cream?*

Various types of creams and ointments may relieve symptoms temporarily, but they do not heal. Actually, it does not really matter which cream or ointment you use, since the therapeutic effect comes from the massage, not from the ointment.

Massage relaxes the muscles, giving the body time to rest and harness its natural healing power. Massage speeds up the circulation, thereby relaxing the painful muscles and raising the body's energy level, which helps the body heal itself. The only objection you may have to ointments is the smell.

e. *Medicines*

I prefer not to interfere as far as medication is concerned. One can't blame a person seeking relief or "breathing space" from unbearable pain. At the same time, one should differentiate between harmful and non-harmful medicines. Dangerous medicines such as Voltaren, which can damage the digestive system, should be avoided. Herbs such as Hypericum or Harpagophytum (Devil's Claw) are recommended. Consult an expert on whether to use a tincture or an infusion and for the correct dosage.

f. *Back support*

During a severe attack, when every movement is painful, wearing a brace will alleviate pain, prevent cramps, and also warm your back a little. Braces should not be used over long periods, even if they feel good, since the muscles become flabby. After recovery, use a brace only when you are exerting effort, in cold weather, or when you feel that the problem is starting up

 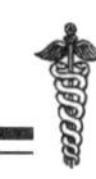

again.

When driving, I recommend using an orthopedic back support, which can easily be attached to the driver's seat. The way you get into the car is important. Rather than getting in feet first, you should sit on the edge of the seat with your feet out of the car. Gently edge yourself into the car, and then bring both feet into the car together. Once you are in the car, move the seat close to the steering wheel to relieve pressure on your feet. When getting out of the car, simply reverse the procedure. First place your feet outside the car, and then follow through with your body.

The back support can easily be dismantled and used in your office or study.

In addition, get yourself a footrest, preferably with an inclined surface, so that your knees will be slightly higher than your thighs, again preventing undue pressure on the vertebrae of the lower back.

g. *Exercises*

As already stated, exercises should be done only once the initial acute stage is over. Again, this varies from person to person. Just as there is no one single type of backache there are no fixed exercises or fixed rules of when to start them. Even two attacks experienced by the same person are not identical.

As a general rule, start with easy neck or back exercises, such as alternately tensing and relaxing the muscles or bending the body from the waist. Begin with five minutes of exercise two or three times a day. As your back improves, you can exercise for up to half an hour. **Never** exercise beyond the pain threshold. As soon as you feel pain, stop. If the exercise itself is painful, skip it.

The following exercises are helpful.

1. Lie on your back on the carpet with your knees bent. Swing your knees gently to the left and then to the right. Continue swinging them from side to side for a few minutes. Separate your knees a little, and repeat the exercise for several minutes, breathing rhythmically.

2. Lying on your back with bent knees, raise one knee to your chest, and then the other. Clasp both knees. While clasping your knees, gently move your lower back, breathing in and out. This is a good exercise, and the carpet will massage your back.

3. Lying on your back with your knees flat against the carpet, stretch your legs with your big toes pointing toward your head, and then relax. Repeat for five minutes.

Complications

If you don't try to relieve the pain and prevent a recurrence, each acute attack of pain could be worse or last longer than the previous one. The pain comes and goes, comes and goes, until finally it comes and doesn't go so easily. After a while, you may experience numbness in your hand or foot, or their muscles may atrophy, leading to a weakness in the extremities. Sometimes the numbness may alternate with acute sensitivity, pain, and cramps. Frequent or recurrent muscular cramps may cause the muscles to harden. This, in turn, can lead to curvature of the spine (scoliosis) or distortion of its natural "S" shape, restricting movement in the upper extremities and making it difficult to walk up and down the stairs.

Prevention and treatment

An attack of pain is a warning signal. There is no need to adopt the fatalistic attitude of some doctors who say: "There's nothing we can do," or "You'll just have to learn to live with it," or "Grin and bear it." Although the anatomical changes in your back may be irreversible, there are many things you can do to relieve the pain and improve your quality of life.

Dieting: Although I am not a dietician, there is no doubt that extra weight makes matters worse. By losing weight, you will alleviate pressure on the spine, legs, and knees. There are many diets to choose from, and you should choose the one that suits you best.

Start by reducing your intake of bread, sugar, salt, and coffee (all of which retain fluids), milk (retains phlegm), and sauces (appetite enhancers).

Avoid	Why?	Acceptable Substitute
Caffeine	Stimulant	Herbal teas, hawayij,* grain coffee, ginger, cinnamon
Processed Foods	Harmful chemicals	Whole grain flours, breads, cereals, crackers, meals
White Sugar	Harmful chemicals	Molasses, maple syrup, honey
Dairy products	Create mucous	Soy or almond milk, almond butter, tofu
Salt	Causes fluid retention	Lemon or potassium salt

*Yemenite mixture of spices.

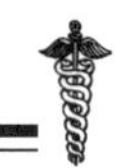

You may also take vitamins, such as the vitamin B complex, but consult an expert first. Shoots, brewers' yeast, nuts, almonds, sunflower seeds, and whole-wheat products are rich in vitamin B.

A 20-minute walk before going to sleep will help you lose weight. (The section on "Overweight" has more suggestions.)

Swimming: Swimming is a useful exercise, but do not overstrain yourself or jerk your head out of the water. You should do some warming-up exercises before entering the pool. After leaving the pool, dry and cover yourself immediately, and then do some heat-generating exercises. Swimming on your back is preferable to swimming on your stomach.

Be careful how you lift and carry things: When lifting things from the floor, crouch instead of bending over, holding the object close to your body. When carrying baskets or bags, divide the weight equally between both hands. Have purchases delivered whenever possible.

Reflexology: Press along line 15, from 45 to 48 and from 13 to 38 (Figure A).

Exercising: During an acute attack, you should not exercise, but once you are on the mend, start with extremely simple exercises, as described above, and proceed gradually to more strenuous ones (walking, stretching, and bending). Be sure to stop as soon as you feel pain. Pain causes the muscles to contract, whereas the whole point of the exercises is to relax the body and muscles. (See Chapter VII for spe-

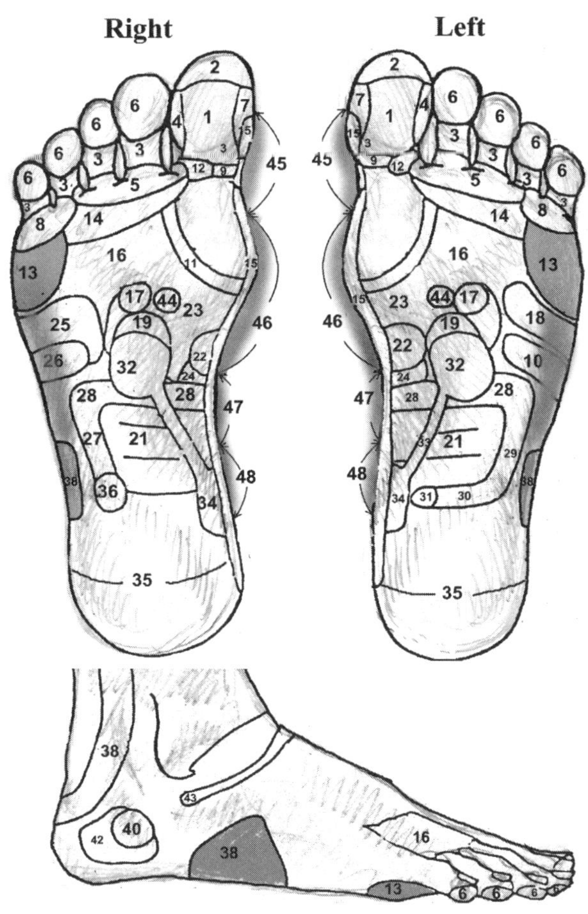

Figure A

cial exercises: for neck and shoulder exercises, do B 3–9; for lower back exercises, do C 1–9.)

Acupressure and Shiatsu: These are ancient Chinese and Japanese methods of relieving pain and releasing blocked energy, through exerting pressure on points (acupressure) or meridians (shiatsu) that control specific areas of the body.

One might argue that since pain is a warning signal, it is beneficial and should not be eliminated. This is not true. In the long term, pain is harmful and leads to muscular spasms. By alleviating the pain through acupressure, we are restoring the body's equilibrium, thereby helping the body to heal itself. So, although the pain is an important signal, once we get the message, the pain no longer serves a useful purpose. On the contrary, it may actually be harmful.

Acupressure points: Of the many relevant acupressure points, I recommend the following five main points: One in the back, one in the thigh, one in the knee, one in the leg, and one in the ankle. These points not only are a representative sample of the most commonly affected areas, but also influence these areas by a process of "remote control."

Back point 1

These points lie on either side of the spine, about two fingerbreadths away from the spine. The points are level with the bottom edge of the ribs (Figure 1).

Back point 2

These points lie behind the hip joint. Since they are located at some depth below skin level, press and knead the area quite hard.

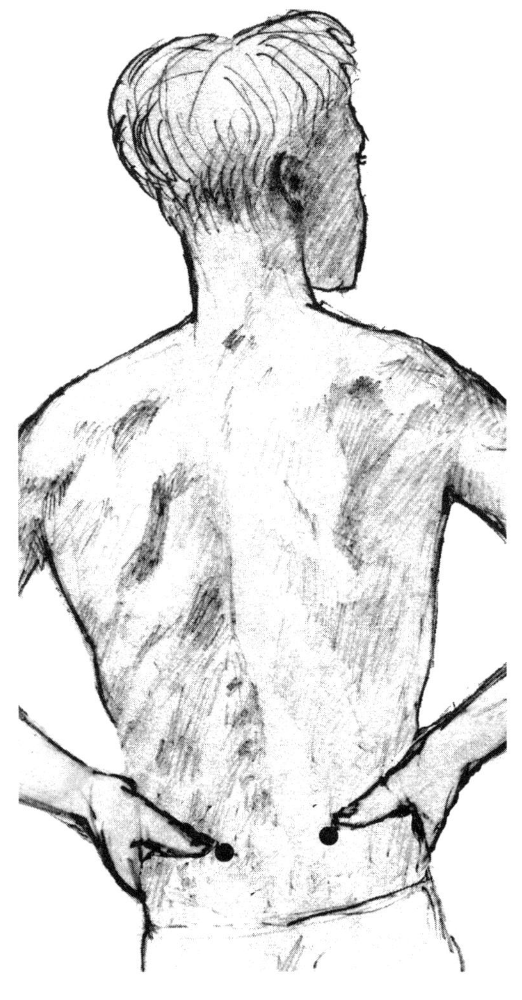

Figure 1

48

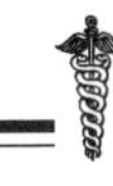

These points are effective in reducing inflammations of the thigh muscle and in relieving lower backaches (Figure 2).

Knee point

The point lies in the center of the fold at the back of your knee (Figure 3).

Leg point

The point is situated in the lower half of the calf muscles (at the back of the leg), at the cross-section of the leg's horizontal and vertical axis (Figure 4).

Ankle point

The point is situated in the depression below the outer ankle. Exerting pressure at this point alleviates lower backache (Figure 5).

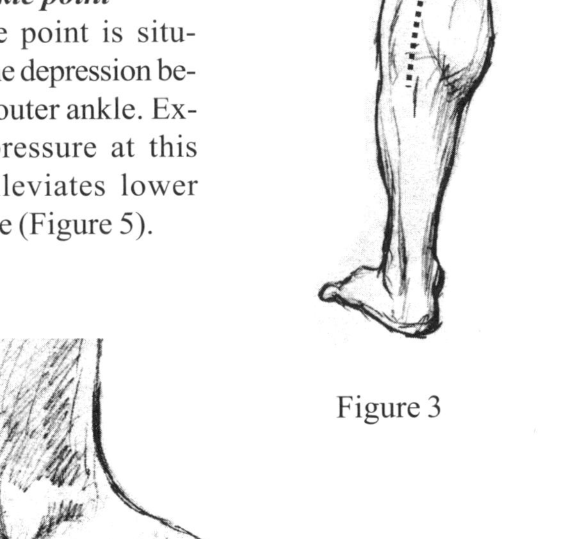

Figure 2

Figure 3

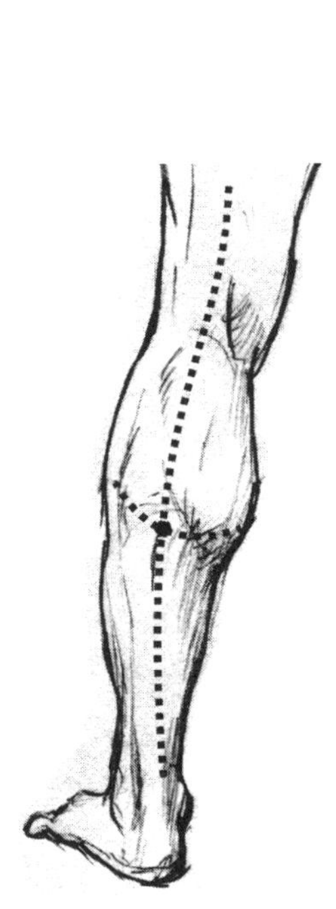

Figure 4

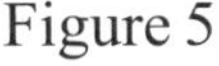

Figure 5

Bone and Joint Pain

Chronic aches and pains in the joint areas usually affect not only the bones, but also the connective tissue between the bones and the muscles; the tendons and ligaments. Typical symptoms include swelling, stiffness, and a sensation of coldness in the painful areas resulting in a lack of mobility in the affected joints. These kinds of problems are particularly common in – though not limited to – the elderly, and are often aggravated by cold and damp weather.

Western medicine has different names for disorders that fit this syndrome including rheumatoid arthritis, gout, etc. Though the cause of these disorders is not clear, it is most commonly thought that the problem lies in the body's autoimmune system. This means that the body's ability to defend itself from harmful outside influences such as cold or bacteria is impaired, resulting in the formation of excess acid that accumulates in the joints and causes problems. Acids and toxins also accumulate in the body as a result of incorrect nutrition.

Traditional Eastern medicine claims that the pain and immobility are caused by psychosomatic causes, or by a blockage of matter and energy. This blockage causes not only localized and radiating pain, but also a sense of fatigue and weakness, which can lead to depression and despair.

Some suggest that the complexities of aging are the determining factor causing these disorders, which are extremely common among the elderly. Others claim that the stress and tension of modern life is the major contributing factor. Yet others blame the widespread inclusion of processed foods into our diets, introducing preservatives, additives, artificial colorings and flavorings, and assorted other chemicals into our bodies.

All of the above claims may have varying degrees of relevance. However, most authorities agree that an accumulation of fluids, matter, acids, and toxins in the joints is what causes the pain and immobility. Therefore, the long-term goal – and by no means an easy one – is to eliminate and attempt to prevent the formation of these toxins.

I recommend a three-fold program comprising diet, exercise, and lifestyle perspectives to help with these types of problems. The suggested treatment options help reduce pain and discomfort.

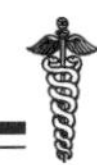

Diet

With joint pain, the primary dietary concept to remember is to avoid foods that produce excess phlegm/mucous and acidity. In general, the body neither absorbs nor excretes these substances and they accumulate in the joints, causing the symptoms described.

Foods to avoid include:

♦ Dairy products – the human body does not absorb dairy products and the mucous that dairy products produce simply accumulates in the joints

♦ White, processed flour – the processing removes important components

♦ Tomatoes and eggplant – these foods produce acids

♦ Animal fats – produce mucous and result in an accumulation of fats

♦ Sugar (and its derivatives) – causes fluid retention

♦ Salt – causes fluid retention

♦ Coffee and tea – cause fluid retention

Reduce your intake of:

♦ Potatoes and peppers – aggravate the problem

♦ Proteins – produce mucous

♦ Oranges – produce acid

Exercise

In general, any gentle exercise that is not stressful to the joints is useful for loosening up the joints and improving your over-all state of health. In particular, I recommend relaxed walking for short distances and swimming. These are both good techniques to get your body moving without unnecessary stress to the joints. Be careful when walking not to use force, and when swimming not to raise your head in an extreme manner. Remember to avoid chills and dampness, as they can aggravate your condition. Cover yourself with a large, dry towel immediately upon leaving the pool and dry yourself quickly to avoid getting chilled. (For special exercises, see Chapter VII: hands, B 1–2; neck and shoulders, B 10–11, B 15–19; knees and ankles D 1–5, D 11–12.)

Recommended foods

Just as a poor diet can weaken the body's resistance, a properly formulated diet can strengthen the body and even alleviate existing symptoms. Following is a table of suggested food substitutes to help you replace harmful food substances with more neutral ones.

Harmful Foods	Suggested Substitute
Coffee	Bamboo, Hawayij* for coffee
Tea	Herbal teas
Salt	Lemon salt, potassium salt
Sugar	Molasses
Meat	Sea fish, turkey, skinned chicken
Dairy products	Soya milk, tehina, almond milk
White flour	Whole grain flours, cereals, breads, grains

*Yemenite mixture of spices. Different mixtures are used for soup and coffee.

Other useful foods to include in your diet, in abundance, are:
♦ Vegetables, particularly broccoli, lettuce, and cabbage
♦ Fruit, except for oranges and persimmons

Lifestyle

Stress takes its toll on all aspects of our wellbeing and the challenge for most of us, no matter what symptoms we are suffering from, is to reduce the level of stress in our lives. There are many steps that can be taken in this direction. Some of the most basic include:
♦ working in a field that is satisfying to you
♦ engaging in leisure pursuits or hobbies that you find pleasant
♦ spending more/meaningful time with your family
♦ reducing/eliminating unnecessary hustle and bustle
♦ simplifying your life
♦ fostering a positive outlook on life

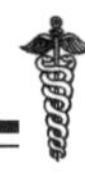

Treatment Options

In addition, the following treatment options may help reduce pain and discomfort.

☐ Hot Compresses
1. Put 1 teaspoon Epsom salts (magnesium salt) into a cup.
2. Add S cup of boiling water and allow it to cool somewhat.
3. Soak a strip of gauze or material in the boiled salt water and place it on the painful area.
4. Leave the compress on until it cools completely, soak again in the hot water, and reapply. Do this for half an hour.
5. Repeat 2–3 times a day.

☐ Sea Baths
Add sea salt to your regular bath water. (Coarse salt can be used instead if you can't get sea salt.)
1. Pour a package of sea salt (available at pharmacies) into the empty bathtub.
2. Add boiling water until the tub is j full.
3. Add cold water until the water temperature is bearable.
4. Soak in the bath for 20–30 minutes.
5. Rinse yourself in clear water (do not use soap).
6. Get out of the bath carefully, it can be slippery, and dry yourself well.
7. Rest for S hour.

☐ Dry Heat
This includes dry sauna, therapeutic mud, paraffin compresses, etc. Most hotels and health clubs have a sauna near the swimming pool. After sitting in the dry heat of the sauna for 10 minutes, jump into the pool or take a cold shower. This is invigorating and refreshing. Therapeutic mud can be bought in a pharmacy. Spread the mud on the affected joints, as directed on the package. Wait until the mud dries and then wash it off. The minerals in the mud have a therapeutic affect.

Warning: People who suffer from high blood pressure or heart problems must consult a doctor before hot sea baths or dry heat.

❑ Herbal Remedies

A mixture of Harpagophytum (Devil's Claw), Hypericum (St. John's Wort), and Chamomile can be quite effective in reducing joint pain. Consult your herbalist for the combination of herbs that is best for your particular symptoms.

❑ Reflexology

First give yourself a general massage, then press along line 15 from 45 to 48, and then from zones 13 to 38 (Figure A).

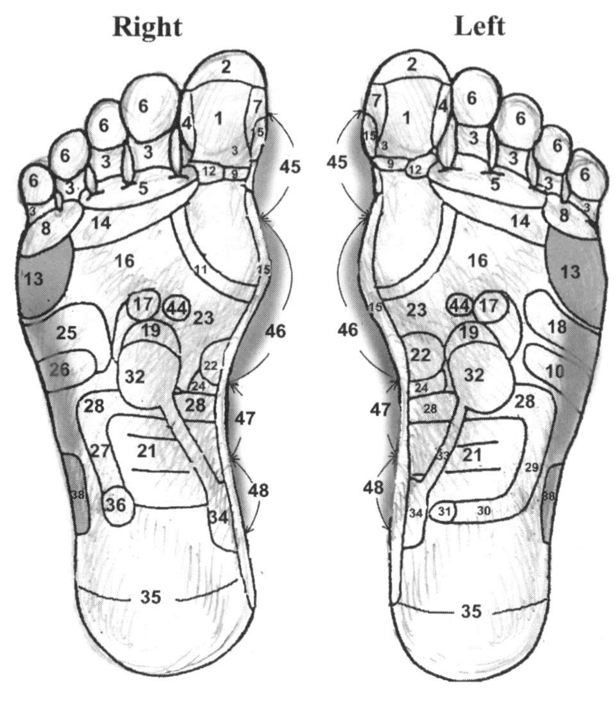

Figure A

❑ Acupressure

Here are two general techniques you can do yourself to help reduce pain in joint areas.

♦ Gentle kneading and massaging of the muscles surrounding the painful joint helps open up various blockages by breaking down the matter that has accumulated. This increases nourishing blood flow to the area. Always work cautiously around painful/swollen areas. Start with gentle pressure and increase the pressure slowly, stopping before it becomes uncomfortable.

♦ Apply firm finger pressure to the "Sea of Energy" acupressure point, which is located approximately two fingerbreadths directly below the navel.

The majority of joint problems occur in the elbows, wrists, ankles, or knees. Here are the recommended general acupressure points for each of these areas.

For a painful **elbow**, hold the elbow with your good hand. With your

54

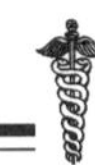

thumb, feel for the tip of the fold made in your bent arm on the outside of the elbow.

Once you find the spot, the elbow should be bent as you apply the most pressure you can tolerate while massaging in a circular motion (Figure 1).

For a painful **wrist**, apply similar pressure to the point located on the wrist, the sniff point, in the depression at the base of the thumb (Figure 2).

For painful **knees**, exert pressure on the small hollow located in the outer part of the kneecap when the knee is bent slightly (Figure 3).

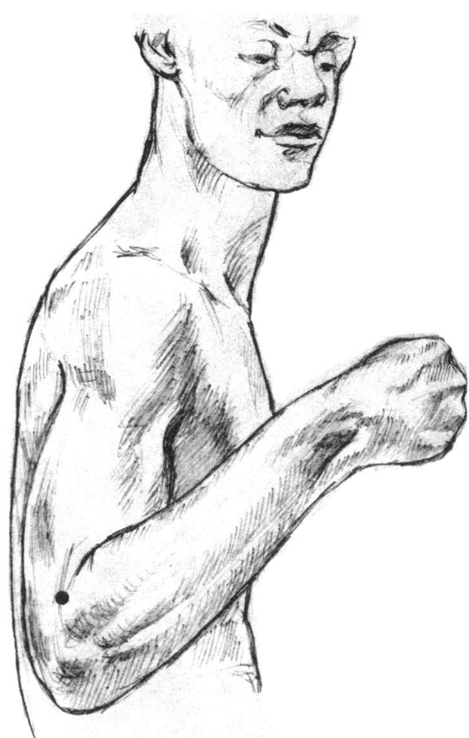

Figure 1

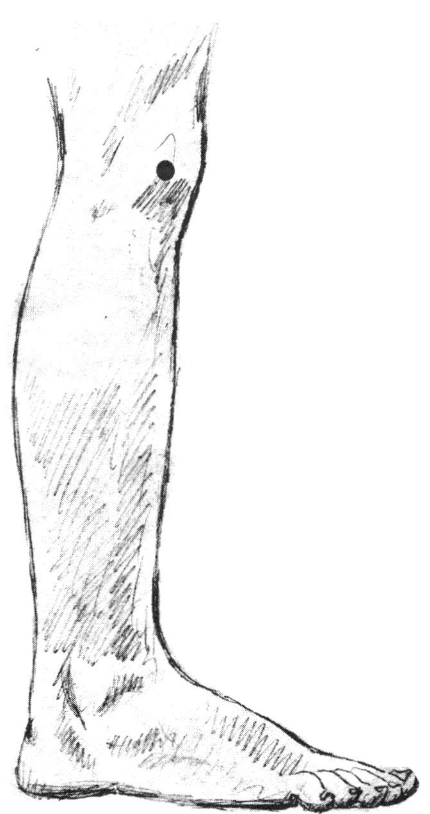

Figure 3

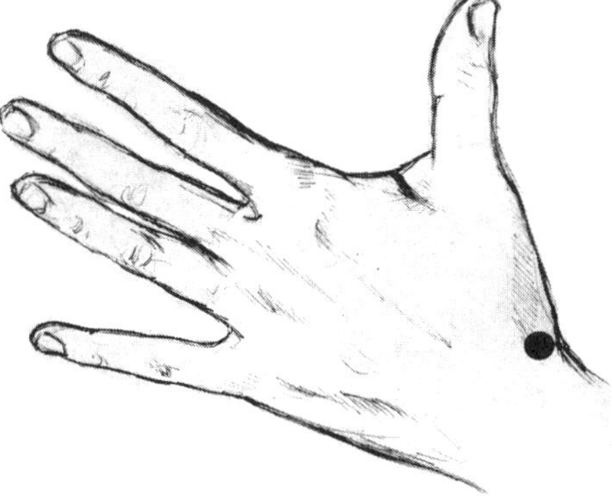

Figure 2

For a painful **ankle**, exert pressure on points located around the ankle (Figure 4).

☐Chinese Massage

Rub clockwise with your palm around the painful joints. Rub briskly to generate some heat and friction. This encourages mobility of the joints, increases circulation, stimulates general body energy flow, and helps move stagnant energy (Figure 5).[1]

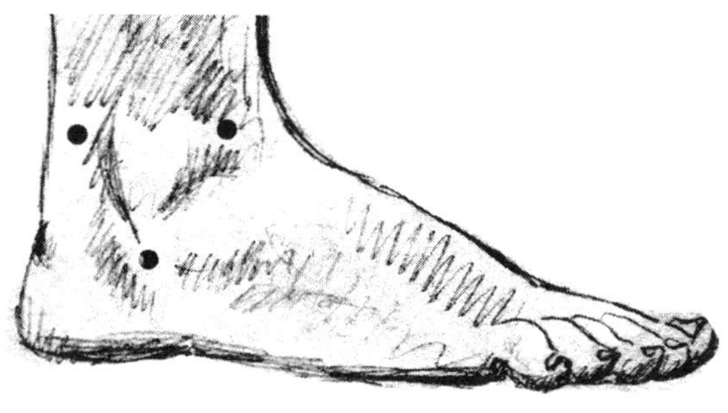

Figure 4

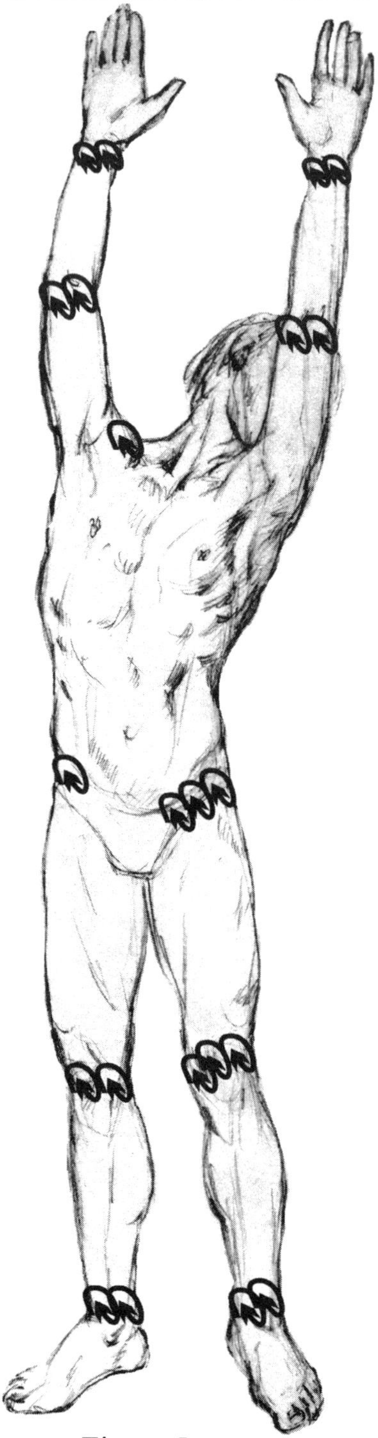

[1]Russell and Gordon, pp.74–75

Figure 5

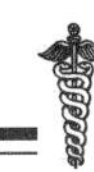

The Common Cold

Every winter people catch colds. They wake up one morning with a runny nose, cough, headache, fever, and aches and pains throughout their body. The cause is not known for sure. Some say it's a virus, others say it's caused by a draft. In any case, the underlying hypothesis is that the body is attacked by some external factor that activates its defense system. You can help eliminate the "intruder" by fortifying the body so that it generates its own cure.

Natural remedies

Rest, changing your eating habits, and drinking a lot are recommended.

Your body needs to rest. Resting helps strengthen the body's natural resistance. Fasting is also helpful. Instead of energy being 'wasted' on digesting food, it can combat the cold. Obviously, by fasting we don't mean a Yom Kippur-type fast, but simply eating less or just drinking.

The food we do eat should be rich in vitamin C. Vitamin C is plentiful in kiwis, red and green peppers, broccoli, parsley, guavas, strawberries, citrus fruit, cabbages, lychees, mangos, and horseradish.

Drink a lot to compensate for the loss of fluids. If you are feverish, drinking will help you perspire, thereby lowering your temperature. Drink mainly herbal teas, such as Chamomile, Cinnamon, Eucalyptus, Thyme, Mint, Sage, Cloves, Ginger, etc. These herbal teas fortify the body so that it can fight the cold.

Cinnamon has a warming effect and therefore diffuses heat. Ginger promotes perspiration, thereby lowering fever.

Eucalyptus, Thyme, and Mint are very good for the respiratory system.

Garlic and Propolis are also effective. Echinacea tincture is a wonderful tonic that strengthens the body's immune system. Recent research shows that this plant helps prevent colds.

If you have a runny nose, add oil of Eucalyptus to a bowl of boiling water. Spread a towel over your head, the upper part of your body, and the bowl, and inhale the steam carefully. Humidifiers are also helpful.

Fever is one of the body's ways of fighting a cold. However, high temperature can be harmful. If your temperature rises above 39 degrees Centigrade, it must be brought down. This can be done by mixing half a cup of alcohol with half a cup of water. Soak a wad of cotton in the solution and spread it over your forehead, chest, stomach, and back. Repeat this each time your temperature tops the 39 mark.

To treat a cough, prepare an onion and honey mixture. Scrape one medium sized onion into one large spoonful of honey. Stir well, strain, and take 2–3 teaspoonfuls, 4–8 times a day.

At night, before going to sleep, rub your chest with olive oil and sprinkle coarse cooking salt over the oil. Spread thin nylon sheeting or a newspaper over it, and put on a warm undershirt. This old folk remedy is extremely effective against coughs and over-production of mucus and phlegm.

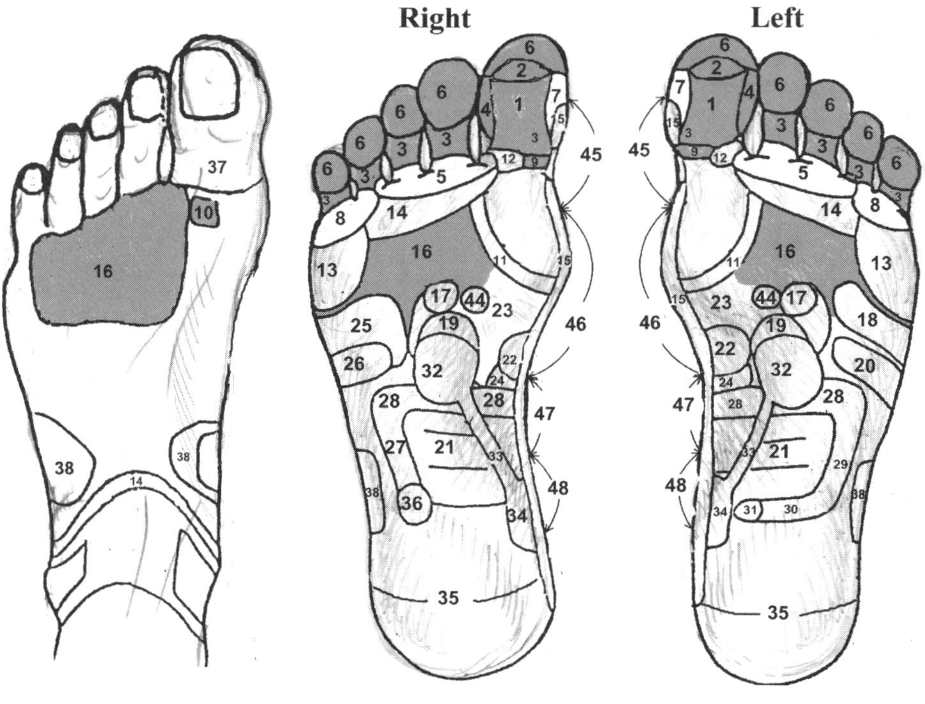

Figure A

Reflexology

First give your feet a general massage. Then massage zones 1,2,3,4,6,9,10 and 16 (Figure A).

58

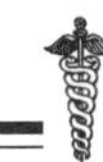

Acupressure

For blocked or runny nose: Press the spots adjacent to the nostrils on either side of your nose. Other points are the middle of the upper lip, and between the eyebrows (Figure 1a, b, c).

For sore throats and general aches and pains: The point is located on the upper part of your hand, just below the mound formed by the junction of thumb and index finger, between the two bones. With your thumb, press down as hard as you can in the direction of the inner bone (Figure 2).

For coughs and breathing problems: This point lies on the inner side of the wrist (Figure 3). The point lies two fingerbreadths away from the fold of the wrist.

If your cold persists, consult a specialist in Chinese medicine. Windcupping (cups placed on the skin that increase the flow of blood by creating a vacuum) and possibly moxybustion (application of heat to the affected area through the combustion of Moxa, a Chinese plant) may be effective. Herbal teas may also be suggested, and a hot water bottle can provide temporary relief.

After you are over your cold, continue eating food rich in vitamin C and taking garlic, Propolis, and Echinacea. Do exercise A 1–7 and B 3–9, from Chapter VII daily.

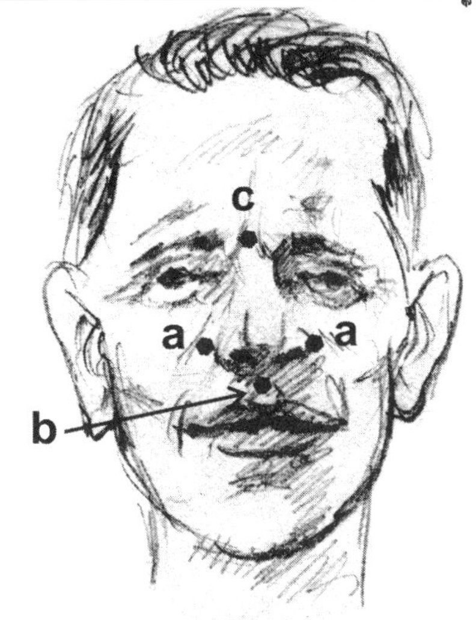

Figure 1

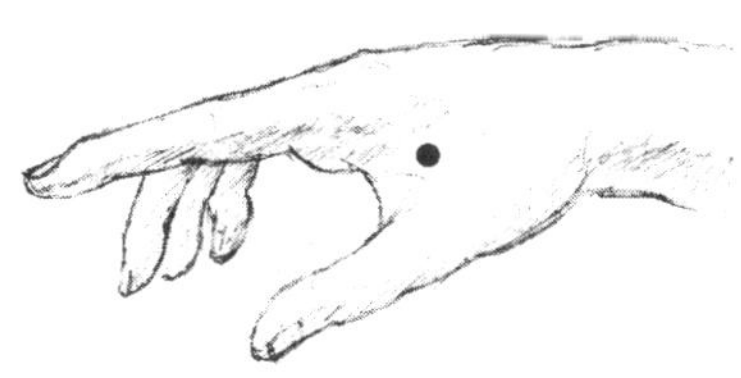

Figure 2

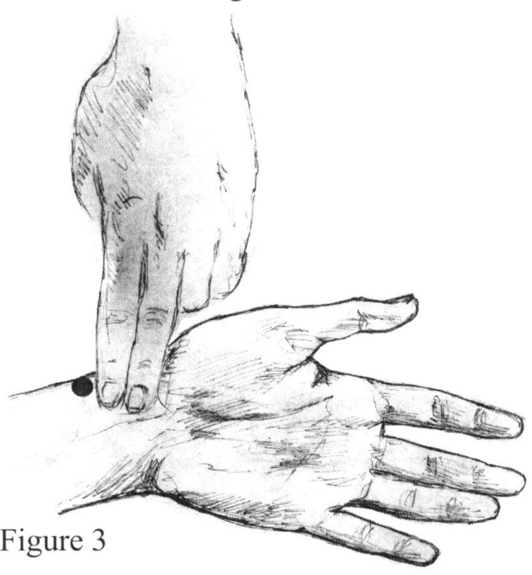

Figure 3

Constipation

Once a young woman came to my clinic complaining of headaches, gas, and nausea. When I asked her if she had regular bowel movements she answered, "Sure, I go to the bathroom once a week. If there is any problem, an enema usually does the trick." Admittedly, this is an extreme case, but it does indicate how little people know about constipation.

Constipation is irregular or inconsistent evacuation of the bowels. This usually means no bowel movement for two or three days, or longer. Normal bowel function means at least one bowel movement a day. Ideally there should be three bowel movements a day.

Regular evacuation of the bowels depends on efficient peristalsis - the rhythmic movement of the muscles lining the walls of the intestines. As these muscles contract and release in an undulating motion, they push the food through the intestines until the unabsorbed waste arrives at the rectum, where it is stored until evacuation (Figure A). When this rhythmic muscular motion is slowed down or weakened, for any reason, the unabsorbed waste

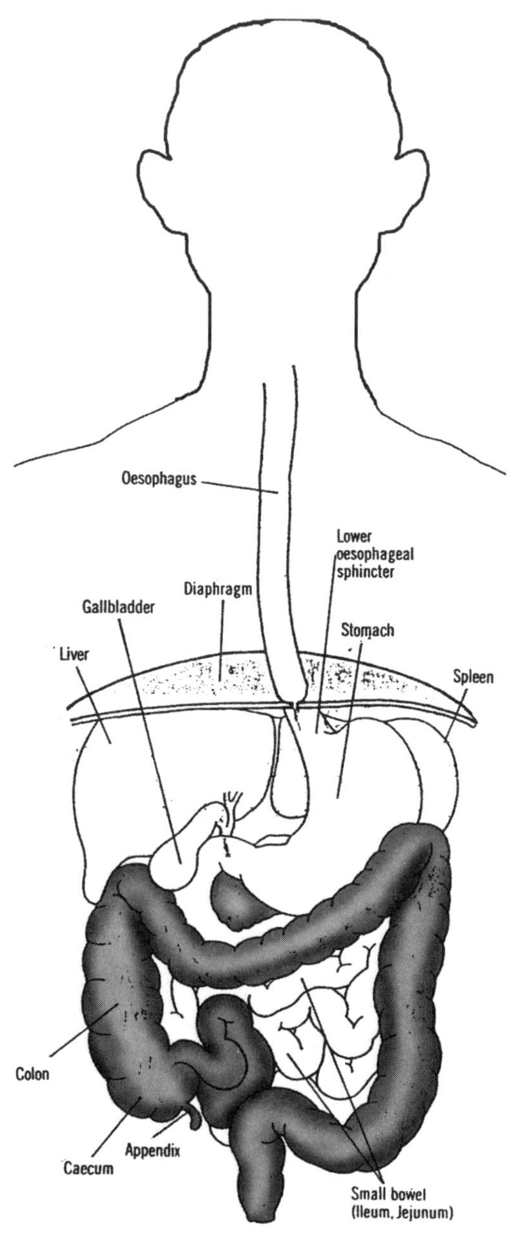

Figure A

60

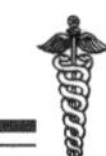

remains trapped in the intestines and the result is constipation. The effects of constipation can include gas, nausea, headaches, and hemorrhoids.

There are a number of reasons why constipation occurs, such as inappropriate eating habits, poor diet, lack of exercise, tension, stress, or not going to the bathroom when necessary. Constipation can also be caused by general weakness as a result of prolonged illness, childbirth, or old age.

Any measure that helps prevent constipation can also serve as a cure. If you are already constipated, apply any measures you decide to use both consistently and strictly.

Prevention

♦ Develop proper eating habits. Eat regular meals, chew your food thoroughly, and stop eating before you are stuffed.

♦ Exercise regularly. Relaxed walking is highly recommended and a moderate pace most closely mimics the body's natural rhythm. Exercises C 3–8 in Chapter VII are especially helpful.

♦ Relaxed breathing. For five minutes every day, lie on your bed with legs bent. Breathe slowly and rhythmically, using your hands to press down on your stomach as you exhale.

♦ Reflexology. Give your feet a general massage. Afterwards, press zone 23, then 21. Continue pressing along the right foot from 36–28, and along the left foot from 28–31 (Figure B). These points correspond to the large intestine.

♦ Proper diet. Eat plenty of fruit and vegetables and natural, whole-grain cereals (brown rice, whole

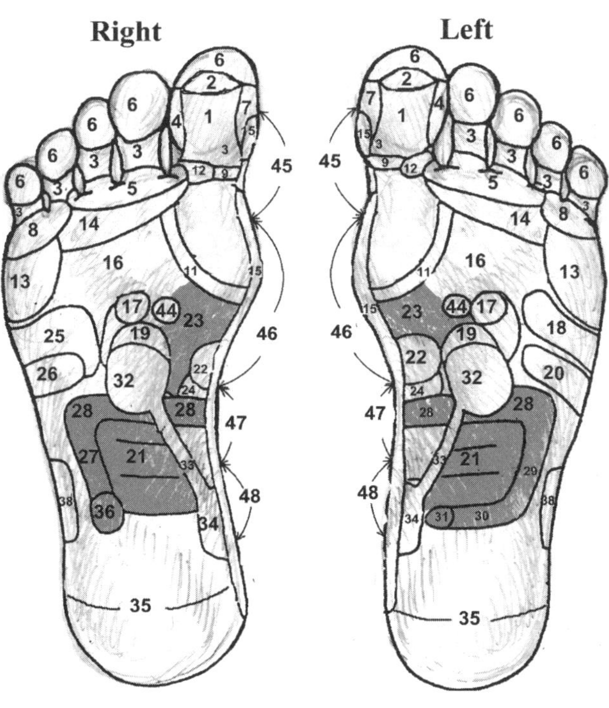

Figure B

wheat bread, etc.) and drink plenty of liquids. Your evening meal should be light, mostly vegetables - particularly lettuce. Include oats in your diet.

◆Regular elimination. Try to train your body functions by going to the bathroom at the same time each day. This is best done in the early morning between five and seven, when bowel activity is at its peak.

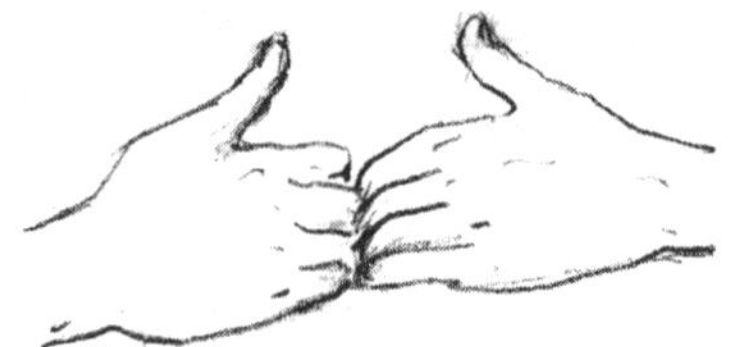

Figure C

Treatment

The suggestions for prevention are also helpful for treatment.

Shiatsu

Use this self-help treatment to stimulate peristalsis.

1. Press down, with four fingers, along the center line of the stomach as you exhale. Start just below the ribcage and continue until just below the navel. Look at Figure C for proper hand position.

2. Continue pressing with four fingers and move to the right following the path of the ascending colon to just above the navel on the right side of your abdomen (Figure D).

3. Proceed left to the other side of the belly and then move down in a straight line towards the left groin.

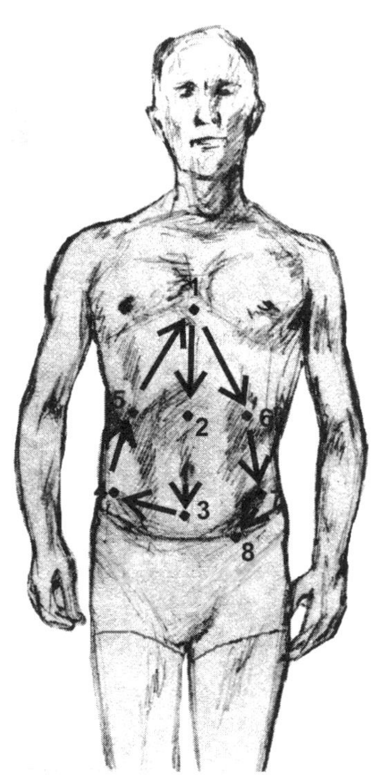

Figure D

4. While doing this take deep, relaxed breaths. Position your fingers as you inhale and exert pressure only when exhaling.

5. Try shiatsu when you are on the toilet. The more pressure, the better the result. Use a footstool for your feet.

Chinese Massage

Following the same principal outlined above, massage the stomach with a large clockwise motion, using warm oil. This helps stimulate peristalsis (Figure D).

62

Acupressure

Apply acupressure at each of the following three points. Press each point five times in succession, for about five seconds each time. Stop. Repeat again and again. Repeat the entire procedure again and again.

◆Located in the soft tissue about four fingerbreadths below the lower edge of the kneecap and one fingerbreadth from the outer edge of the shinbone (tibia) (Figure 1).

◆Located on the outer part of the lower arm, four fingerbreadths up from the wrist (Figure 2).

◆Located just below the anklebone on the inside of the foot. Find the point and then continue pressing all along your instep until you reach the root of your big toe (Figure 3).

Dietary Recommendations

◆Vegetables, especially those high in fiber such as lettuce, cabbage, celery, beet root, and cooked carrots.

◆Fruit, especially apples (with the peel). But avoid guava, banana, pomegranates, quinces, sabras, and persimmons.

◆Whole grains such as rice, wheat, legumes, and beans.

◆Try foods from the following list and see what works best for you: watermelon, pineapple, bamboo shoots, cherries, millet, olive oil, lettuce, eggplant, mustard, turnips, apricots, Swiss chard, crab apples, chicory, grapes, papaya, green peppers, coconut, squash, garlic, sesame, plums, dandelions, loquats, dried fruits, strawberries, corn-on-the-cob, tamarind, yams, asparagus, barley, oats, onions, pears, pumpkin seeds, raspberries, and soy beans.

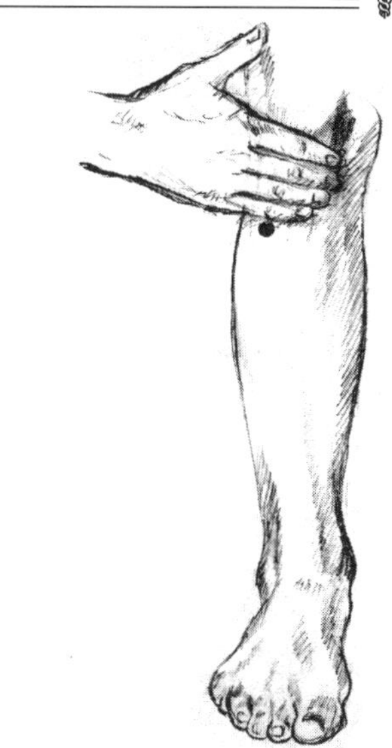

Figure 1

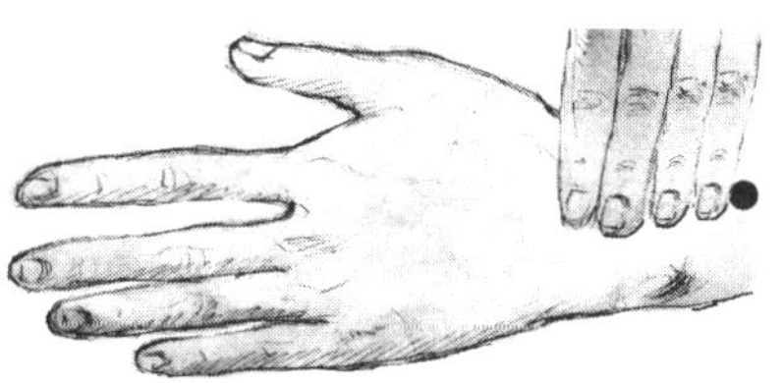

Figure 2

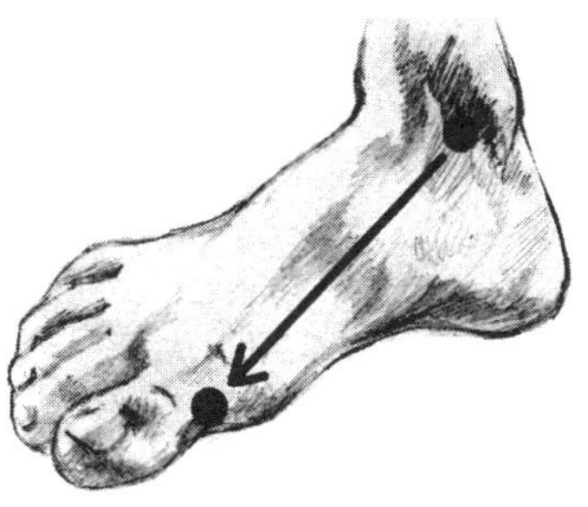

Figure 3

Other remedies

♦ Soak dried fruit overnight in water. Drink the water in the morning.

♦ Eat seaweed mixed with water before breakfast.

♦ Stir 1 tablespoon of bran into a container of yogurt. Drink 2 cups of water after eating the yogurt-bran mixture. Drinking the water is necessary; otherwise, the constipation will become worse.

♦ Drink tomato juice in the morning, on an empty stomach, followed by a cup of hot coffee.

♦ Fasting every few days is a good way to clean out toxic waste from the body. Fasting has the same effect as an enema.

♦ Herbal formula: make an infusion from 20 grams each of the following herbs, which can be purchased at a health food store:

Frangula (Buckthorn) -	Diuretic
Salvia (Sage) -	Demulcent
Plantago (Plantain)-	Diuretic
Taraxacum (Dandelion) -	Laxative

Place a teaspoon of this herb mixture in a cup. Add boiling water and let steep for ten minutes. Strain and drink the tea. Honey can be added.

♦ Soak Linseed seeds overnight and eat the jelly that forms with yogurt or sour cream.

♦ Scrape a teaspoon of Aloe Vera leaf jelly into half a cup of cold water. Mix and drink.

♦ Use a juice extractor to extract the juice of an Aloe Vera leaf, add honey and drink.

♦ Drink, drink, drink. Cold water, hot water, water with honey, water with table salt, water with Epsom salts, grapefruit juice, milk, spinach juice with sour cream, lemon juice with olive oil, a mixture of equal amounts of celery, carrot, and beet juice. See what works best for you.

Do not take laxatives. They weaken the body and aggravate constipation in the long run. If there is no other choice, use an enema or take Cassia (infusion) or sea kelp (seaweed) once, never on a regular basis.

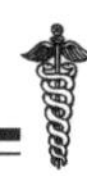

Diarrhea – A Dangerous Nuisance

Diarrhea is frequent or very frequent movement of the bowels. The feces are usually watery and diluted, and sometimes contain undigested food. There are two types of diarrhea, acute and chronic. Acute diarrhea occurs all of a sudden and lasts for a limited period of time. Chronic diarrhea is a constant condition.

Diarrhea is one way for the body to eliminate toxins or spoiled food. Vomiting is another. Eating too much, eating food that is too cold, eating fruit or drinking fruit juice can also cause it. Other causes of diarrhea can include irritability, anxiety, allergies, colds, flu, antibiotics, and other medications.

Though most often it is an uncomfortable nuisance causing stomach aches, cramping, and general debilitation, diarrhea can be dangerous due to the loss of body fluids, important substances, and "good" germs that help our digestive system. Babies and young children can become dehydrated. (See "Diarrhea" section in Children's Ailments, Chapter IV.)

Remedies

Prevention of diarrhea involves proper eating habits, regular meals, a suitable and varied diet, and a calm way of life. If you're already afflicted with diarrhea, reduce your food intake and start drinking. Herbal teas such as Mint, Sage, and Chamomile are particularly effective against diarrhea, as is blueberry juice.

For acute diarrhea, seep an ordinary tea bag in a quarter cup of boiling water for a few minutes. Then empty the contents of the bag into the liquid and drink it, tea grains and all. The grains cause the stomach to contract and this stops the diarrhea. Pomegranate juice is another effective remedy and boiled pomegranate peel is even better. Simply boil the peel in water for a few minutes, and then drink the water after discarding the peel.

Diet

The first thing you should do is rinse out your stomach with rice water. Boil the rice (1 cup white rice to 7 cups of water) on a low flame until it turns into a gelatinous mass. Strain it and drink the liquid. The next day, you can add a little salt to the rice or mix it with yogurt. Bananas, toast, and

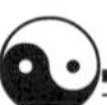

cooked carrots are also effective.

Reflexology

Massage the left foot from 31 to 28. Afterwards massage the right foot from 28 to 36 (Figure A).

Chinese Massage

Using olive oil, massage the stomach with counter-clockwise motions. Massage in this direction helps to slow down hyperactive peristalsis (intestinal contractions), which is what causes diarrhea (Figure B).

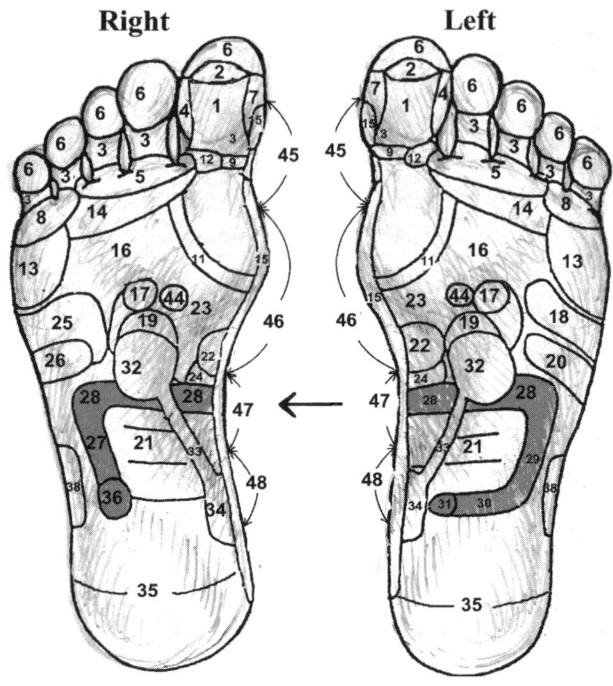

Figure A

Herbal Remedies

This herbal formula will eliminate stomach acids that aggravate chronic diarrhea. Use 20 grams of each herb.

Filipendula (Meadowsweet) - Astringent.
Uva Ursi (Blueberries) - Astringent.
Quercus (Oak bark) - Astringent.
Fennel - Excellent against gas.
Chamomile - Absorbs gas.

Put 1–2 spoonfuls of the mixture into an empty cup and add one half cup of boiling water, seep for ten minutes, filter, and drink the tea. If it is too bitter, you may sweeten the tea, but do not use honey, which usually acts as a laxative.

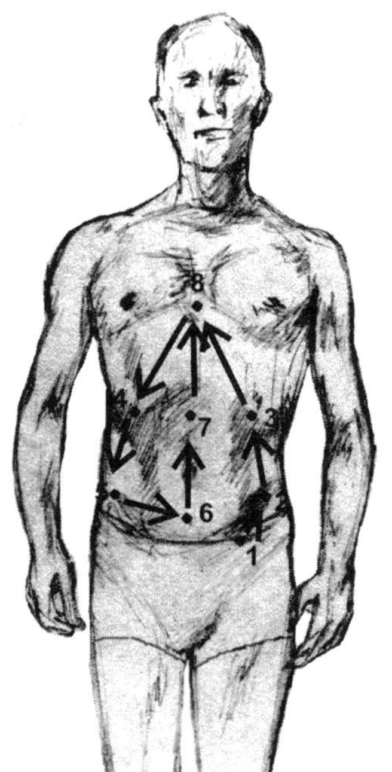

Figure B

66

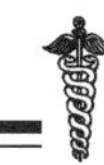

Acupressure

These acupressure points help stop diarrhea. Try any or all of them.

1. Colon point #11 is located at the edge of the external fold of the arm that is created when your elbow is bent (Figure 1).

2. This point is located at the base of your toe on the inside of your foot. Start applying pressure at this point and then keep pressing along your instep until you reach the bottom of the ankle (Figure 2).

3. This point is located on the hand between the first and second bones. Apply pressure with your thumb in the direction of the second bone of the hand (Figure 3).

4. This point lies about 4 fingerbreadths below the knee-cap, 1 fingerbreadth along the tibia toward the outside of the leg. Apply pressure from either a seated or reclining position. Use your thumb to apply pressure in a downward direction, then massage with upward motions (Figure 4 – next page).

5. This point is located on the

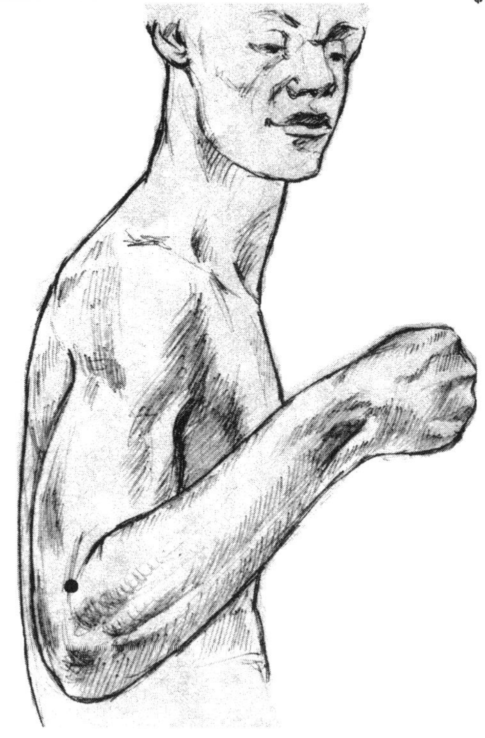

Figure 1

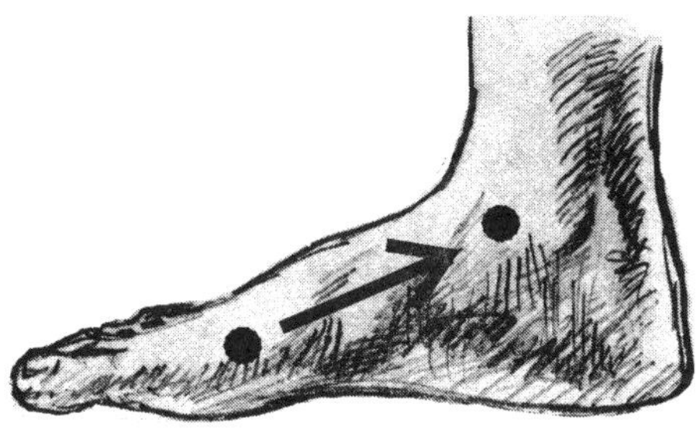

Figure 2

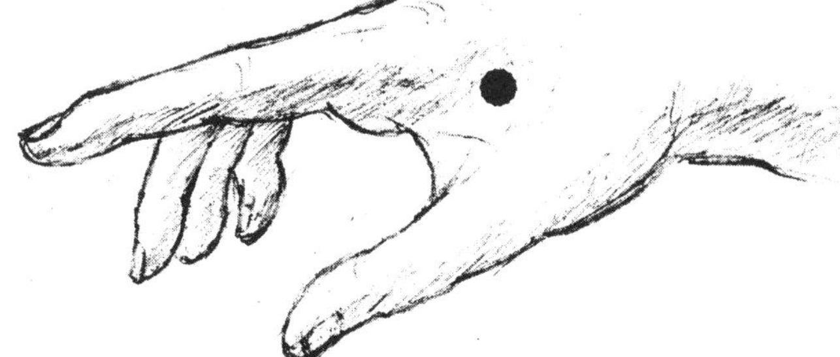

Figure 3

stomach, about 6 fingerbreadths directly above the navel. In a sitting or reclining position, use your thumb or palm to massage inward, towards the body (Figure 5).

6. This pair of points lies about three fingerbreadths from the navel on either side. Apply pressure and massage in a counter-clockwise direction to slow down bowel movements (Figure 6).

7. This point is located precisely on the navel. Pinch and massage the navel in a counter-clockwise direction. Continue massaging with your finger in a counter-clockwise direction.

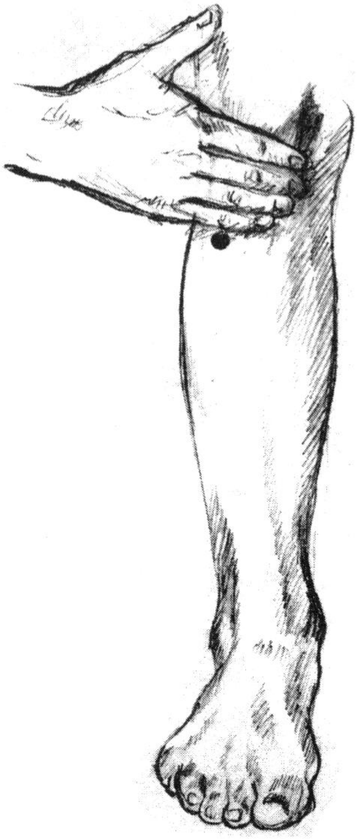

Figure 4

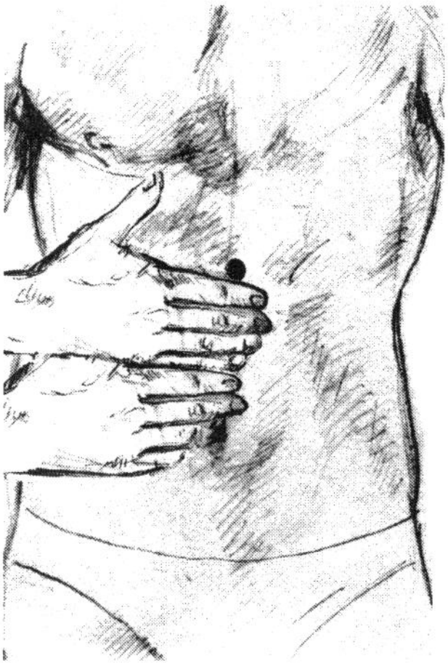

Figure 5

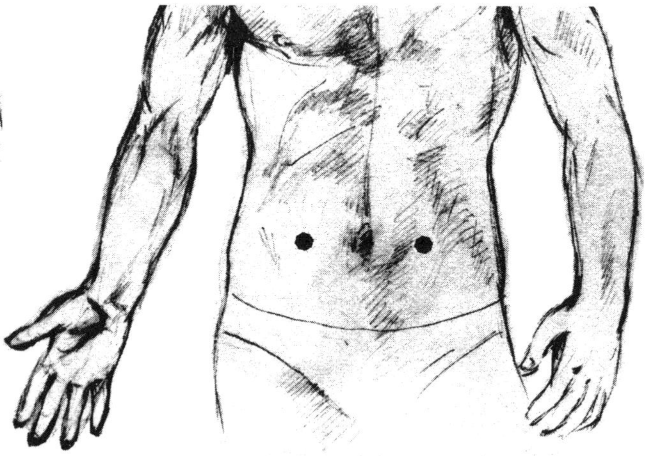

Figure 6

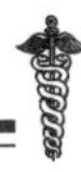

Headaches

If the ancient Chinese doctors would hear commercials on the radio or television, they would be incensed by the sweeping statement that one tablet can cure everything: "Got a headache? Take acamol. Got a sore throat? Take acamol. Got a toothache? Take acamol."

Chinese medicine not only differentiates between a headache, a sore throat, and a toothache; it also differentiates between the various kinds of headaches, each of which represents a different problem. Treatment therefore varies, depending on the problem. What this means is that a headache is not itself an illness, but a symptom that something is wrong.

According to Chinese medicine, the head is a sensitive area because it is the meeting point of the meridians that pass through the hand or leg to the head, or that leave the head for the body (meridians are channels in the body through which energy flows).

The body may be attacked by external factors (what the West calls viruses or bacteria) or internal factors (such as toxins in the blood due to faulty diet, "moodiness" and tension, or incorrect breathing). These factors disturb the flow of energy and blood into the head and cause a blockage or stoppage in the meridians and veins that pass through the head. According to Western medicine, the headache results from a constriction or dilation of the blood vessels in the head or a chemical change resulting in the above.

The Chinese call a headache that is triggered by an internal factor a "head wind." They do not mean a "dybbuk" that is trying to escape from the head! Rather, they are referring to a severe, recurrent, and uncontrollable headache, which seems to be triggered by tension or defective functioning of various organs.

Diagnosis

In Chinese medicine, headaches are diagnosed by whether they result from a situation of "surplus" (acute headaches) or "deficiency" (chronic headaches).

In Western terms, "surplus" denotes an acute attack, in which young and generally healthy people are affected by an external factor beyond their control, such as wind, cold, virus, or bacteria, or an internal factor such as overeating, or eating foods one is allergic to. This can result in a variety of symptoms – including headache. A situation of "deficiency" (chronic headache), on the other hand, denotes a weak person with a low energy level. Such a person may simply have been born with a weak constitution and succumbs easily to each gust of wind (in both the physical and psychological sense). Chronic headaches are typical of adults whose body or organs have become weakened or diseased. When such a person is attacked from within, he is unable to withstand the onslaught, but must rely on divine mercy or on a doctor who can make him stronger and better able to resist or fight the disease.

Note that headaches that are triggered by a "surplus" are different from those triggered by a "deficiency." Headaches triggered by a "surplus" (acute headaches) are characterized by a violent, sharp pain accompanied by dizziness, restlessness, a bitter taste in the mouth, nausea, and a sense of constriction in the chest. Usually, heat and pressure do not alleviate the headache. On the other hand, headaches that are triggered by a "deficiency" (chronic headaches), which are usually caused by weakness and tension, are persistent, but react well to heat and pressure. Other symptoms can include weakness, exhaustion, palpitations, insomnia, a pale tongue, and a weak pulse.

Another important diagnostic factor is the location of the headache. The location helps us trace the energy meridian that is linked to a specific organ. This tells us which organ is not functioning properly and enables us to get to the root of the problem, either by treating the organ itself, or the meridian that connects it to the head.

There are four main locations: posterior

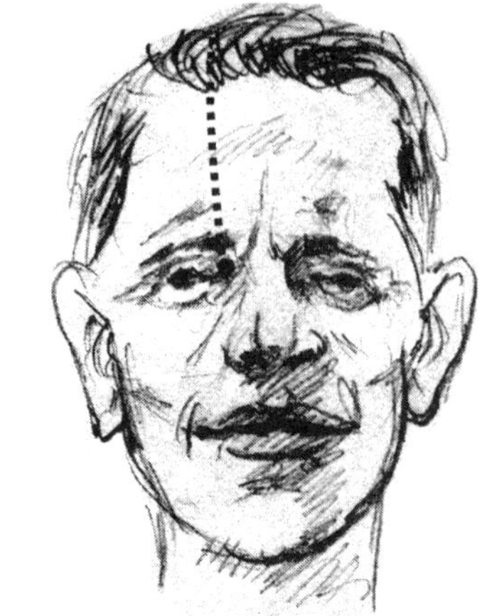

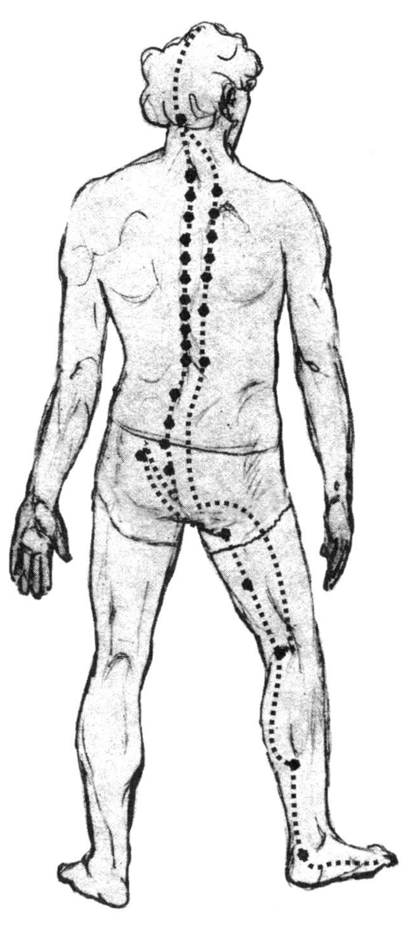

Bladder Meridian
Figure 1

70

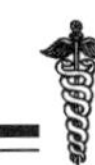

headaches, anterior headaches, lateral headaches, and cranial headaches.

Posterior headaches

These occasionally begin with a back-ache (usually upper backache), with the pain traveling through the shoulder and neck, sometimes radiating out to the fore-head. Such headaches may be connected to torticollis (stiff neck), or colds (exposure of the back of the head to wind, in Chinese medicine). Sometimes these head-aches may appear after an accident with a whiplash effect. Usually posterior head-aches do not move. According to Chinese medicine, if they do move, they are prob-ably headaches caused by exposure to wind or cold. The meridian (a channel in the body that runs beneath the skin and be-tween the muscles, through which energy flows) responsible for posterior headaches is the bladder meridian, which passes along the head and back (Figure 1).

Anterior headaches

If the headache "moves," it is gener-ally symptomatic of an "ordinary" cold. The organs responsible for this are the lungs and bronchial tubes. Such a head-ache is usually accompanied by other symptoms of a cold, such as sneezing, ca-tarrh (mucus in the nose and throat), cough-ing, etc.

Anterior headaches may also be trig-gered by sinusitis, which may or may not result from a cold. These headaches begin at night, so that the person wakes up with a bad headache. He feels heavy and bloated, due to the mucus that has accumulated in

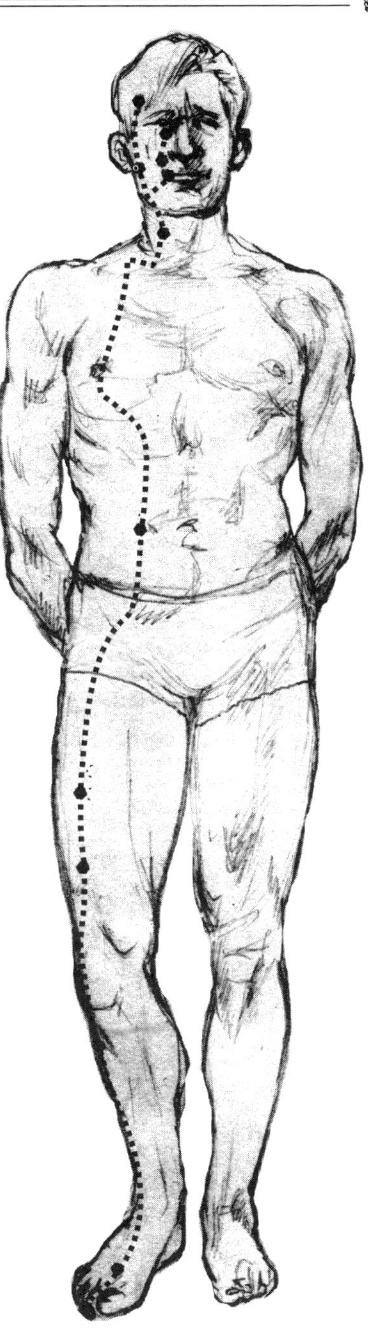

Stomach Meridian
Figure 2

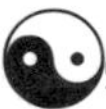

the nasal cavity and the head. Such headaches occur more often when people eat a late supper and then sleep on their stomachs. During the night phlegm and humidity rise from the stomach to the head, causing a headache that sometimes borders on a migraine (see section on Migraines).

Anterior headaches may also be caused by constipation (both chronic and acute). Toxins that are stored in the stomach rise and cause the headache. The situation is aggravated when a constipated person sleeps on an empty stomach.

Another trigger for anterior headaches may be a mild or undetected toothache. Anterior headaches may occur between dental appointments.

Mild anterior headaches that get worse after reading or watching TV may well be connected with the eyes. They tend to occur mainly in middle-aged people and in people who have to switch between regular and reading glasses. Sometimes the headaches occur in people who don't even know they need glasses, or in people whose sight has suddenly deteriorated and who squint to see better, without realizing it.

Anterior headaches are usually not strong, but are persistent and tiring.

The meridian responsible for all types of anterior headaches is the stomach meridian, which begins under the eyes and passes through the face down the chest and through to the feet (Figure 2).

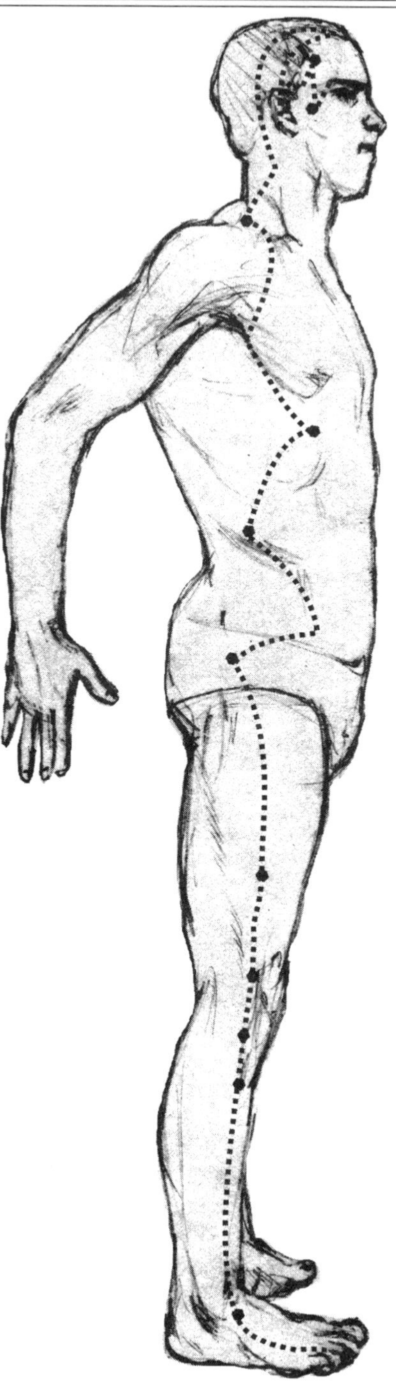

Gall Bladder Meridian
Figure 3

72

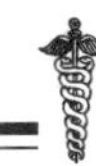

Lateral headaches (at the side of the head)

These are problematic headaches, which usually turn into migraines. They are problematic because they often have a psychological trigger, particularly anger. When a person gets angry, "the blood rushes to his head" through the temples and the eyes, causing a bad headache.

Sometimes, a lateral headache continues for a number of days with accompanying nausea, and leaves the sufferer exhausted (see section on Migraines). A lateral headache may be a symptom of high blood pressure, especially when connected with anger or worry. In such cases, it may turn into a full-blown headache and travel to the cranium (top of the head).

Another lateral headache that can develop into a cranial headache is a menstrual headache. Such a headache may be a symptom of PMS and disappear once the period starts, or begin in the middle of the cycle and continue to the end of the cycle, due to the loss of blood and fluids. Such a headache may also develop into a migraine.

According to Chinese medicine, the meridian responsible for lateral headaches is the gall bladder meridian that encircles both sides of the head twice, descending on either side of the body to the feet (Figure 3).

Cranial headaches (at the top of the head)

This is the most "psychological" type of headache - caused mainly by too much thinking, worrying, insomnia, etc. It may be a direct headache, resulting from tension or

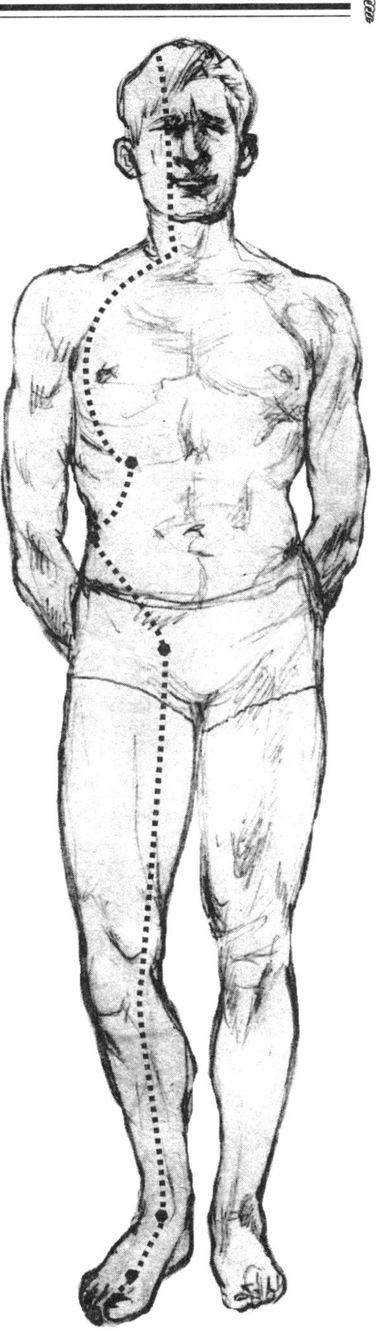

Liver Meridian
Figure 4

"pressure," or an indirect headache, caused by high blood pressure, exhaustion, and sleep disturbances. It may be related to PMS, loss of menstrual blood, or menopausal tension caused by loss of estrogen (see section on Menopause).

A cranial headache can also be caused by low blood pressure or by various illnesses that disturb the blood supply to the brain. A cranial headache may begin with a stabbing pain in the region of the temples, moving to the head. Although cranial headaches sometimes resemble migraines, they do not occur in cycles and are not connected to the season. When it's hot, the headaches usually get worse. In such cases, it is important to drink a lot. According to Chinese medicine, the liver meridian is responsible for cranial headaches. (The liver is the body's largest and most "irritable" organ.) This meridian begins between the first and second toes, and continues to either side of the chest, near the heart, liver, and gallbladder (Figure 4). From the chest, a branch continues to the throat, the eyes, and the top of the head.

Chinese medicine connects the liver with the eyes, which explains the link between eyes and headaches.

Prevention

I would advise everybody who suffers from headaches to read the section on Migraines. Due to the large variety of headaches and their causes, I shall outline two basic approaches:

The holistic approach: This approach combines a healthy diet, herbs, a moderate way of life, and avoiding anything that may cause an imbalance. One should engage in physical activity, have satisfying work, leisure pursuits, a spiritual goal, and a challenge in life.

On a long-term basis, Feverfew can be helpful. This herb also prevents migraines.

The specific approach: As explained above, Chinese medicine diagnoses headaches in terms of "surplus" and "deficiency," blockage of blood and energy flows (or excessive blood and energy flows), exposure to wind and cold, or as the result of external and internal factors.

Above all, the headache is a sign that something is wrong in the body's organs or meridians. Therefore, in addition to the above, preventive measures should also relate to the specific problem.

There are many specific preventive measures and I strongly recommend that you read through various articles to try and find ways of dealing with your specific problem. For example, vitamin C, found in citrus fruit, red peppers, guava, etc., has a strong preventive effect. If the headache may be an allergic reaction – try avoiding foods such as white sugar, white flour, and saturated fats (cookies, sweetened beverages, and chocolate are out). Also avoid dairy and meat products, wheat, corn, and the like (see section on Allergies).

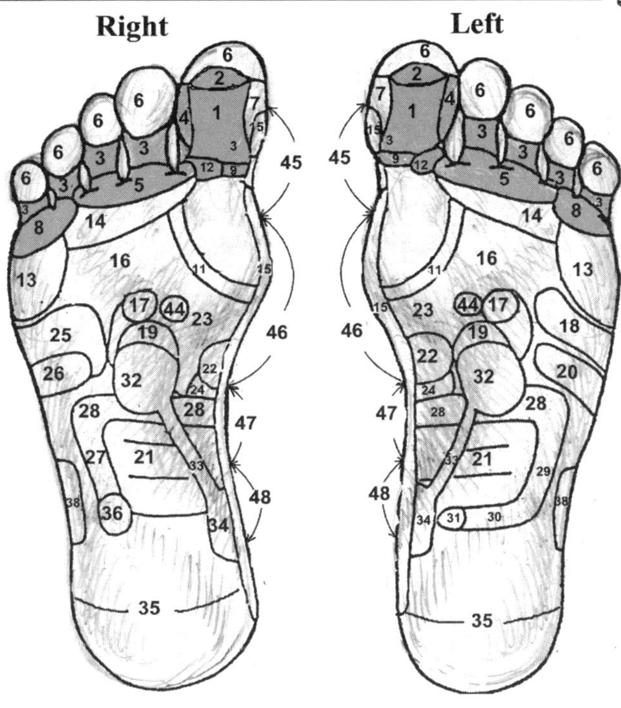

Figure 5

If so many foods are forbidden, what can we eat? Someone once said: "If I were as wise before the event as after the event, everything would be fine." I suggest we be wise after the event, but immediately after. Through a process of trial and error, we can determine which food we are allergic to, which food or drink caused the headache, and omit it from our diet. Eat foods that are rich in calcium, such as sesame, tehina, green peppers, broccoli, lettuce, and above all, drink a lot.

Exercise: Refer to Chapter VII. Exercises A 7 and B 3–9 are especially helpful.

Cure

When in the grip of a headache, apply all the above remedies more intensively.

Take special note of the following:

♦**Reflexology**: Concentrate on the toes and their base: 1,2,3,4 and 5,8,9,12 (Figure 5).

◆**Diet**: Do not eat, but drink as much as possible.

◆**Rest**: Lie down until the worst of the headache is over.

◆**Relaxation, focusing, and breathing**: Lie down and relax. Focus on the headache. Breathe in and breathe out toward the center of the pain. This alleviates the pain and relaxes the body. If the pain moves to other parts of the head, or even other parts of the body, "run after" it and "capture it" by focusing on it. "Running after" the pain and focusing on it can also help us trace the source of the pain, and its itinerary.

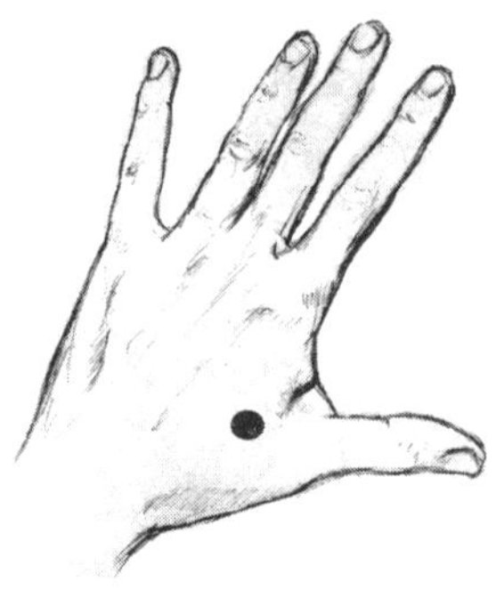

Figure 6

◆**Acupressure**: Use your mind and hands to comb through the entire region of your head. If you manage to trace the pain's path or meridian, begin pressing down along it. Press any part, meridian, or point that hurts. If the pain is acute ("surplus" type), press hard. If the pain increases, stop pressing. If the pain is chronic ("deficiency" type), press gently each time you breathe in and out, or tap light rhythmic taps with your fingers or knuckles. Allow your fingers to massage painful areas on your face, head, and neck.

If you have some knowledge of meridians, and energy flow directions (see Chapter II, An Eastern Perspective, for an explanation of meridian theory), press against the direction of the flow for acute headaches ("surplus"), and with the direction of the flow for chronic headaches ("deficiency").

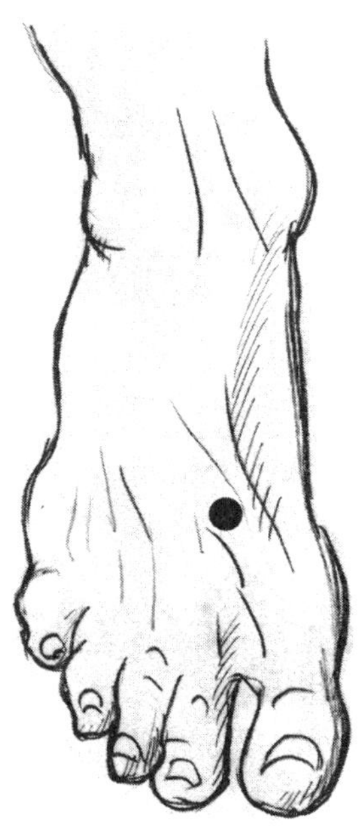

Figure 7

Acupressure points

1. First general point (pain point, or wrist point)

The point lies at the base of the mound formed by the junction of your thumb and index finger. To help you locate this point, place the thumb of one hand between the thumb and index finger of the other hand, as shown. The point is situated at the edge of your thumb (Figure 6).

2. Second general point (foot point)

This point lies on top of the foot, between the continuation of the big toe and the second toe, about two fingerbreadths away from the base of the toe (Figure 7).

Posterior headache

3. Neck points

This pair of points lies one fingerbreadth away from the spine, on both sides and level with the natural hairline. Press both points simultaneously and continue pressing along the back of the head towards the ears(Figure 8).

4. Hand point

This point lies on the side of the hand, one fingerbreadth above the base of the little finger. Bend your hand – the point is where the fold forms (Figure 9). After finding the point, relax and press with your other hand.

Anterior headache

5. Forehead point – relaxation point

This point is located between the eyebrows. Pinch hard with thumb and finger (Figure 10).

6. Hand point – cold and phlegm point

The point lies two fingerbreadths away from the fold of the wrist (Figure 11 - next page).

Lateral headache

7. Temple points

These are two points, on either side of the forehead. Each point is situated in the area of the temple, about one fingerbreadth away from

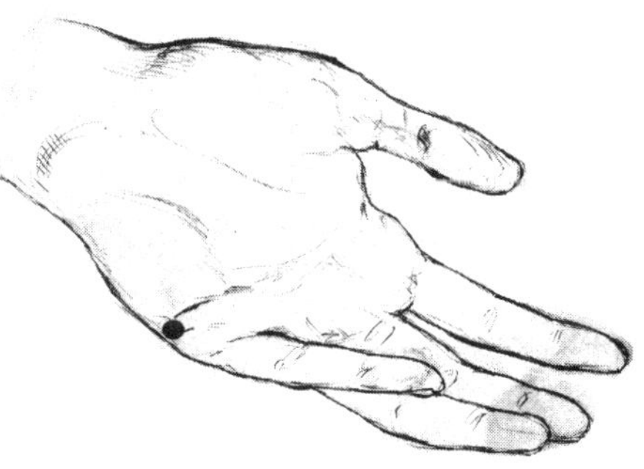

Figure 8

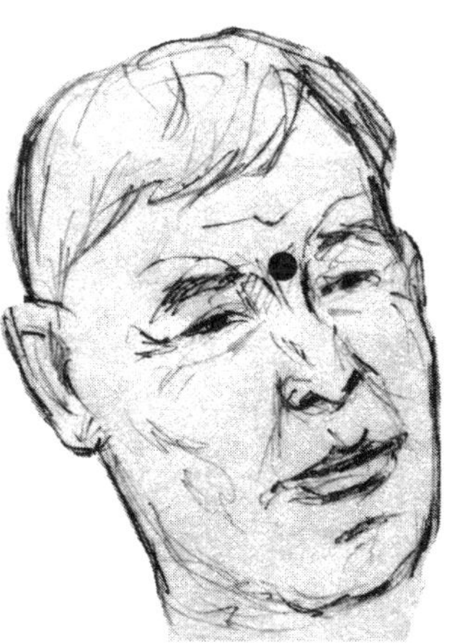

Figure 9

Figure 10

the eyebrows. Press gently, and continue pressing in the direction of the eyes toward the edges of your eyebrows (Figure 12).

8. Hand point

This point lies on the outer part of the lower arm, three fingerbreadths away from the wrist (Figure 13).

Cranial headache

9. Head point – the "thousand junctions" point

This point lies at the junction of the line that rises from the top of the ears and the line rising from the middle of the nose toward the top of the head. Press or tap on this point (Figure 14).

10. Elbow point – point for lowering blood pressure

This point lies on the elbow. Bend your elbow and locate the external fold of the arm. The point lies at the edge of the fold (Figure 15).

In this review of the various types of headaches and their causes, I rely mainly on Chinese medicine. The preventive measures described are based on a natural, Western approach. I suggest ways of treating headaches that rely on self-healing. These methods include drinking, rest, relaxation, focusing, massage, and acupressure.

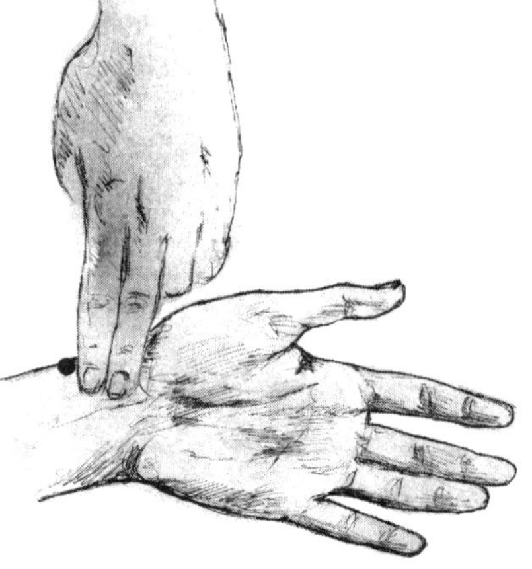

Figure 11

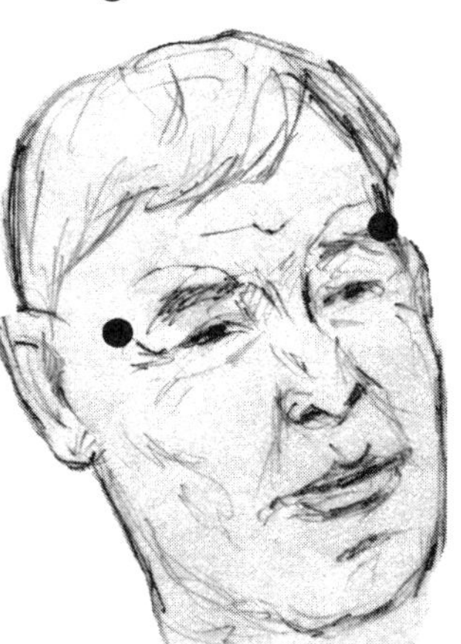

Figure 12

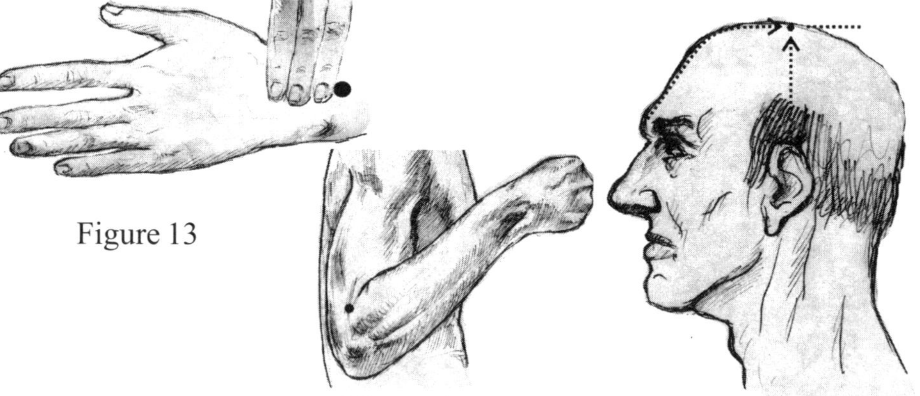

Figure 13

Figure 14

Figure 15

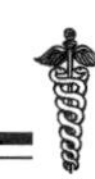

Migraines – A Natural Approach

Migraine is a complex condition that is hard to treat and whose symptoms vary from person to person. Western medicine is unable to cure migraines. Its "solution" is to give the sufferer drugs or tranquilizers and inform him that "it's something he has to live with." Alternative and natural medicine, on the other hand, try to approach the problem in a variety of ways. In many instances, acupuncture and herbal remedies are effective. Chinese medicine, with its holistic approach, tries to ascertain whether the migraine is the result of a "surplus" or "deficiency," stress or weakness, enlargement or constriction.

What is a migraine headache? What are its causes? What are its symptoms? Can it be prevented and if so, how? How can one diagnose the root of the problem? How can it be treated? We shall try to answer these questions.

A migraine manifests itself mainly as a severe headache on one or both sides of the head. It has three stages: the preliminary stage, the full-blown attack, and the final stage. Migraine-sufferers learn to recognize the symptoms of the onset of an attack during the preliminary stage.

The full-blown attack consists of a paralyzing headache with blurred vision, pain in the eye on the affected side, and extreme sensitivity to noise and light. The attack can last from a day to as long as a week in extreme cases. During the attack, the victim feels miserable, restless, and helpless. Family and friends also feel impotent. Nausea and vomiting may accompany the early, middle, or final stages of an attack. Most attacks leave the person feeling exhausted or weak. In some cases there is loss of bladder control. Worst of all, the sufferer knows that although this particular attack may be over, it's not the last.

Attacks usually occur periodically, and may be triggered by a variety of causes. While the onset of menstruation is a frequent cause of migraine in women – tension, food allergies, neck and shoulder problems, or changes in the weather may also precipitate attacks. During these attacks, chemical changes in the body lead to a chemical imbalance in the cerebral (the brain's) blood vessels, causing some of them to contract and others to expand. The expanded blood vessels cause the headache associated with migraine. These chemical changes are also responsible for the related symptoms, such as nausea and vomiting.

Causes

There are various theories that attempt to explain what causes migraines. Most of the theories agree that the immediate cause of the migraine is the expansion of the cerebral blood vessels.

◆ The allergy theory

This theory ascribes the cause of migraine to an allergy. It claims that migraine is a genetic condition, the onset of which usually occurs at a young age although it can be triggered at any age. According to this theory, histamine accumulates in the blood, leading to the dilation of the peripheral blood vessels. The dilation of the cerebral blood vessels is what causes the migraine attack.

Chinese medicine has a slightly different perspective. It claims that surplus matter (e.g., acids, toxins, and phlegm) rising to the head obstructs the blood vessels causing the headache.

◆ The hormonal theory

According to this theory, migraines are associated with menstruation. The onset of menstruation releases a flood of hormones that dilate the cerebral blood vessels, resulting in migraine headaches.

Chinese medicine believes that the migraine is triggered by the accumulation of premenstrual blood. The build-up of pressure prior to menstruation generates heat that rises to the head, causing tension, irritability, anger, bloodshot eyes, and headaches – typical symptoms of premenstrual migraine.

◆ The atmospheric pressure theory

This ascribes migraines to changes in atmospheric pressure – for example, flying or climbing a steep mountain. The rarefied atmosphere causes blood to collect in the lower part of the body. The heart is unable to pump enough blood to supply the brain with the amount it requires. The blood vessels expand, resulting in a migraine headache.

This explanation ties in with the Chinese theory of deficiency, where the depleted blood supply is unable to nourish the cerebral blood vessels.

◆ The impaired liver–metabolism theory

According to this theory, the migraine is caused by impaired liver and gall bladder function. The liver's inability to eliminate toxins from the body leads to a build-up of these toxins in the brain. This, in turn, causes the blood vessels in the brain to expand and causes a chemical fluid to be secreted that triggers the migraine. The Chinese ascribe impaired liver function to stress, repressed emotions, consumption of fatty and "hot" foods, and excessive

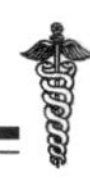

consumption of alcohol.

◆ Shoulder and neck problems

Shoulder and neck problems can also cause migraines by pressing on the nerves that lead to the head, causing the muscles to constrict. The Chinese see these problems in terms of a deficiency. The constriction in the neck and shoulder muscles obstructs the blood vessels in the head, which causes stagnation and deprives the brain of blood.

◆ Stress

Stress causes chemical changes in the brain that result in a migraine. This can be the main cause of the migraine, or a secondary development accompanying most of the other precipitators.

Symptoms

Allergic migraines

Preliminary symptoms include rash, runny nose, sneezing, and sometimes puffiness under the eyes. The pain starts at the top of the head and descends to the eyes, nose, and teeth. At the end of the attack, urine is abundant and dark.

Hormonal migraines

These always begin with dysmenorrhea (painful periods), cramps in the lower abdomen, swollen breasts and abdomen, nausea, vomiting, and shooting pains – usually around the temples. When the attack ends after a day or two, the patient's urine is abundant and dark.

Atmospheric pressure

This type of migraine afflicts people who are affected by climatic conditions and weather changes. Preliminary symptoms include dizziness, apathy, fatigue, and joint and muscle pains. The pain can begin anywhere in the head and move to both sides.

Impaired liver function

This type of migraine always begins with pain in the upper right-hand side of the abdomen, intestinal hyperactivity (flatulence), and nausea. Other symptoms include sneezing and an itchy nose, and pain around the eye. The pain is only on one side - on the right for right-handed people and on the left for left-handed people. The attack always ends with excessive vomiting.

Stiff neck and shoulder

This kind of migraine begins with a torticollis (stiff neck) due to a crick in the neck, an uncomfortable sleeping position, a cold, or whiplash. The actual migraine sets in several hours after the precipitating event. Pain is felt at the back of the head (the parietal region), radiating out to the eye and ear. Symptoms are tearing eyes, ringing ears, and blurred vision or hearing. Paleness, puffiness under the eyes, and a sensation of cold in the body, particularly in the hands and feet, are other symptoms. The attack lasts for several hours. A comfortable position may offer some relief.

Prevention

Migraines are so complex that it is almost impossible to prevent them entirely. However, a good rule of thumb is that anything that improves your health in general will also alleviate the symptoms of a migraine. Correct nutrition, a relaxed way of life, regular exercise, a happy family life, satisfying work and hobbies, a spiritual goal, and a challenge in life greatly reduce the number and severity of attacks. We shall consider these factors in greater detail, and apply them to each type of migraine.

If the migraine is related to menstruation, deal with the problem between cycles when the chances of relief and cure are especially good.

Nutrition: If you suffer from allergic migraines and suspect a food allergy, a process of elimination might establish which foods you are allergic to. Common foods that cause allergies are milk (produces phlegm) and dairy products, chocolate, red wine, fatty (e.g., margarine, fatty meats) and "hot" foods, etc. (see section on Allergies).

All migraine sufferers should have oats and lettuce for supper. These foods are relaxants and will help you sleep better. Sound sleep is important and will help you cope with the problem instead of letting it get the better of you!

Relaxation: A relaxed way of life is especially important in stress-related or spastic neck muscle-related attacks.

Physical exercise: Physical exercise is especially important when the migraine is caused by impaired liver function.

Walking is important. A daily 20-minute to half-hour walk in fresh air stimulates peristalsis (contractions of the intestines), which activates the digestive system. This speeds up the metabolism, helping clear obstructions (including energy blockages) and eliminate the toxins that can cause migraines. (Exercises A 7 and B 3 - 9 in Chapter VII are especially helpful.)

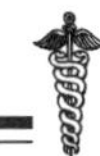

Relaxation exercises are important when cramped shoulder and neck muscles contribute to the problem. Since torticollis (stiff neck) is always present during a migraine, either as a cause or as a symptom, neck and general body exercises are important. Choose simple exercises that can be done at home, for 5 - 10 minutes in the morning, 5 - 10 minutes at noon, and 5 - 10 minutes in the evening (like morning, afternoon, and evening prayers). Deep breathing is very effective. While lying on your back, breath slowly and deeply, in and out. At the same time, slowly move your legs back and forth, rightward and leftward, in time with the deep breathing.

Relaxation exercises, uphill and downhill walking, and breathing are also effective in treating migraines that are caused by changes in atmospheric pressure.

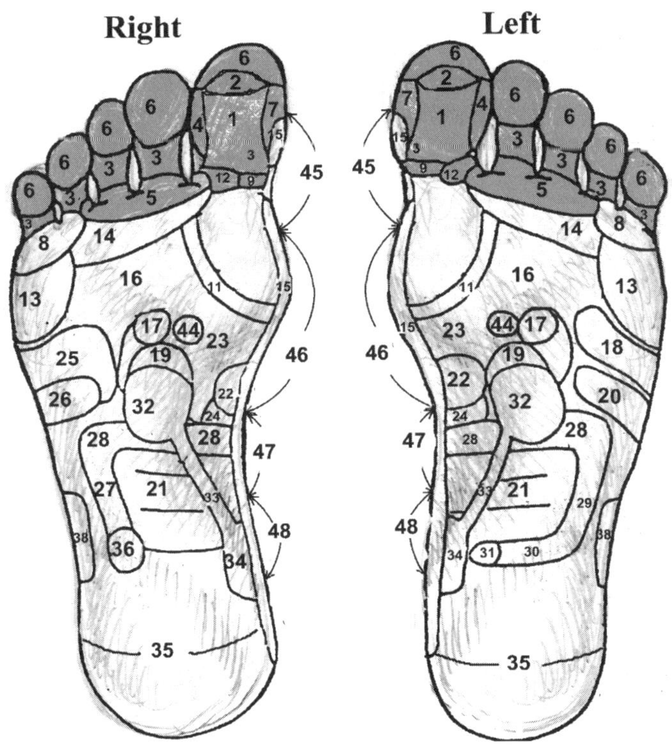

Figure A

Reflexology: Give your feet a general massage. Then apply pressure and knead zones 1,2,3,4,7 and 5,6,9,12 (Figure A). Do this between attacks.

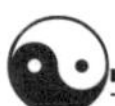

Treatment

In treating migraines, the key word is prevention. Therefore, all the advice given above is part of the cure.

Chinese Massage: Opening the Fan

Apply a little oil to the tips of your fingers. Place each hand over half of the face, thereby covering the entire face. Slide your hands apart, revealing your face (Figure B).[1]

Herbal remedies

Herbal teas such as Chamomile, Sage, Liquorice, and Melissa (and possibly also Rosemary) should be substituted for tea and coffee (although in some cases, coffee actually helps during an attack, since it helps to contract the dilated blood vessels in the head). An herb that seems to be useful in the long term is Feverfew, which must be taken for a long time. Many migraine sufferers find it helpful in the long run, to make the attack shorter and less severe, and to suffer from attacks less often.

Shiatsu and Acupressure

Between attacks, and particularly when the preliminary signs of an attack occur, apply firm pressure to the back of your head, starting with the large depression at the back of your skull (medulla oblongata) and moving out to the sides. Then apply pressure to the neck muscles at the

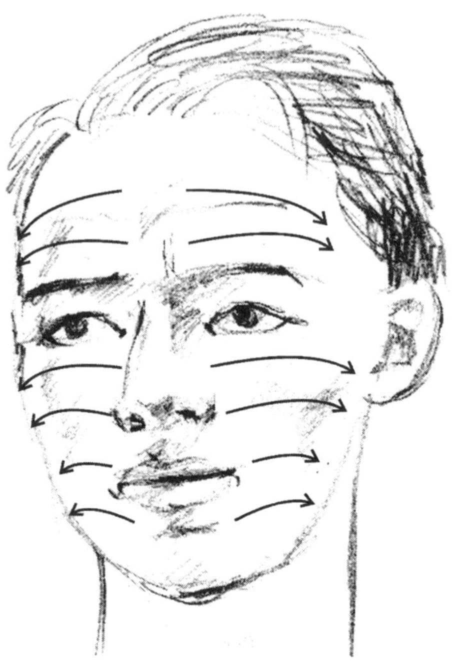

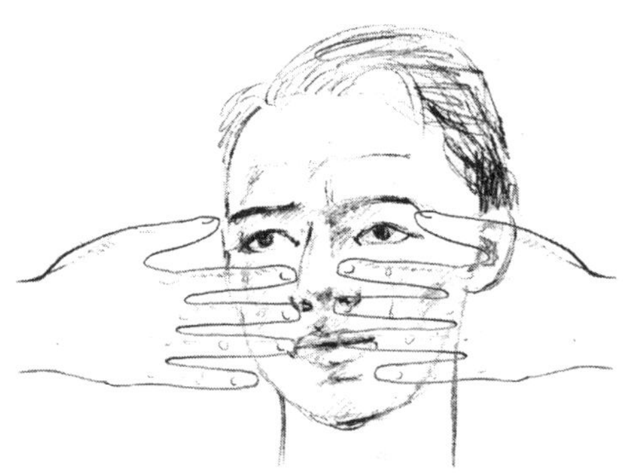

Figure B

84

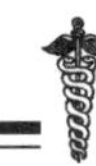

base of your head, moving down toward your shoulders. Finally, ask your partner to apply pressure and massage the trapezial muscles in the shoulders (Figure 1).

For those suffering from impaired liver or gall-bladder function, shiatsu should be applied at the following points: at the base of the foot between the fourth and fifth toes, and between the big toe and the second toe. According to Chinese medicine, these points demarcate the end of the gall-bladder meridian and the beginning of the liver meridian (Figure 2).

The following acupressure points – finger pressure on specific points – are optional:

1. The point mid-way between your eyebrows (Figure 3).

2. The points where your eyebrows begin (Figure 4).

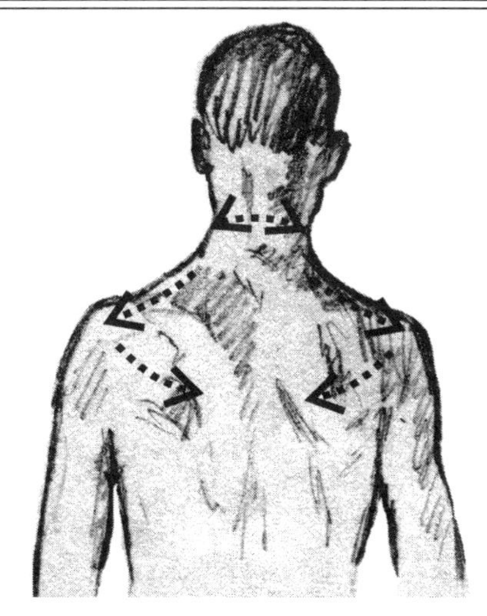

Figure 1

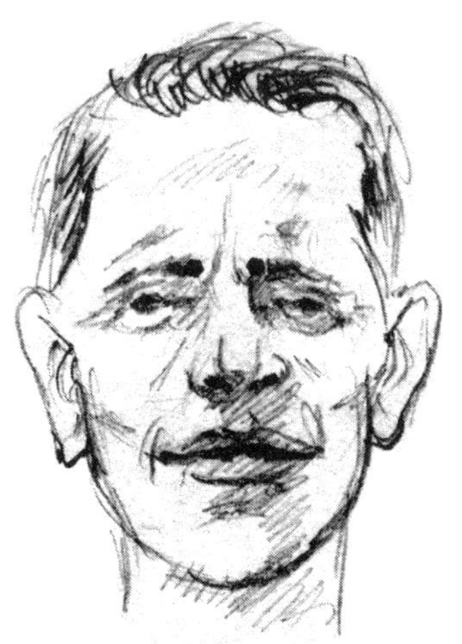

Figure 2

Figure 4

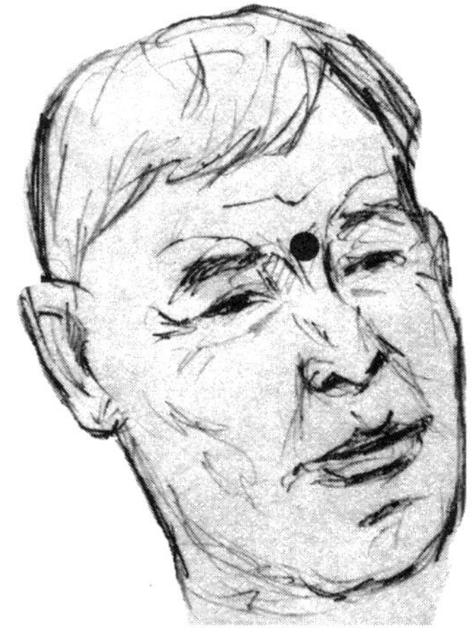

Figure 3

These points are especially effective when sinusitis is present. Also useful in such cases are the two points slightly above and to the sides of the depressions above your eyebrows.

3. The points where your eyebrows end (Figure 5).

4. The points above your temples, about one fingerbreadth away from the edge of the eye socket (Figure 6).

5. The antipain point.

The point lies at the base of the mound formed at the junction of your thumb and index finger (Figure 7).

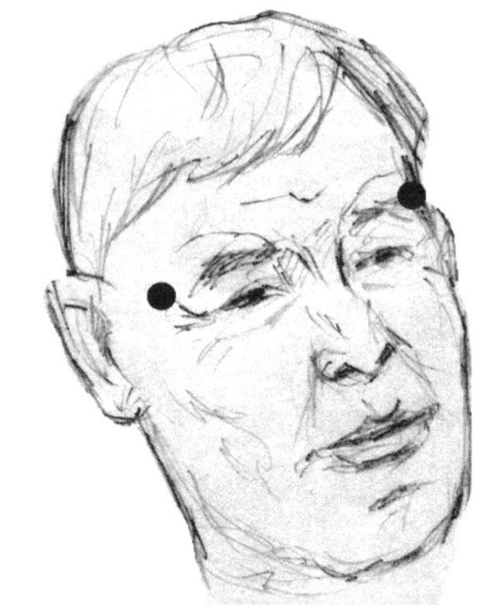

Figure 5

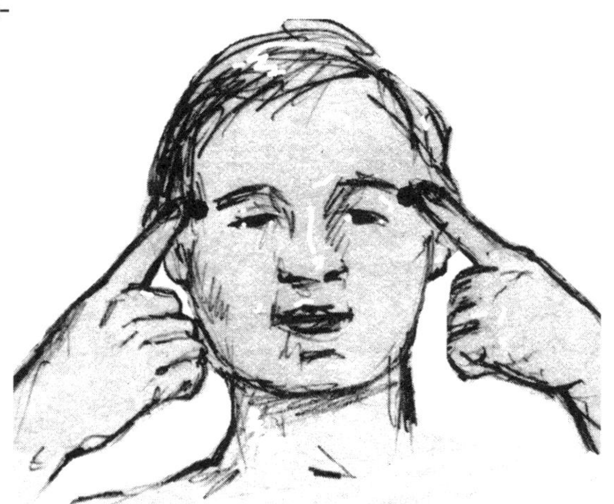

Figure 6

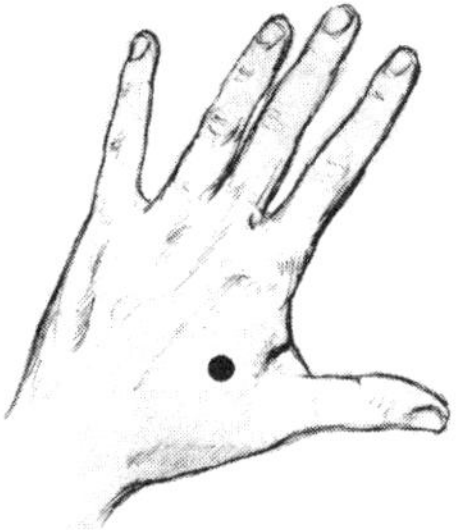

Figure 7

[1]Russell and Gordon, p. 44

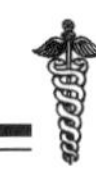

Menopause - the Change of Life

*Written together with Mrs. Chava Stroh, qualified
in complementary medicine.*

During menopause many women suffer a variety of unpleasant symptoms. One of the most uncomfortable is hot flashes accompanied by perspiration. Hot flashes occur in all seasons. Even opening a window doesn't help. Another disagreeable side effect of "the change of life" is anxiety and moodiness. Women who used to be calm and relaxed are now depressed, anxious, and moody. However, the good news is that today there are ways of preventing or eliminating these unpleasant symptoms.

Symptoms

The physical symptoms of menopause include hot flashes, itching, dry skin and dryness around the vagina, and a tendency to put on weight. The psychological symptoms are tension, depression, mood swings, palpitations, and sleep disturbances. Sometimes women decide to make major changes in their lives. Divorce is quite common; the children have grown up and left home, making it possible to divorce without the children suffering. However, the decision to divorce usually has more to do with changes within the woman herself, than with other problems. Although low-level tension may have existed between the couple for years, it is menopause and its attendant changes that usually cause the marital problems to escalate into a crisis. This explains why this period in a woman's life can be referred to as the "menopausal revolution."

The most serious menopause-related medical problems are high blood pressure, heart attacks, and a tendency to develop osteoporosis (a loss of bone mass). Osteoporosis can lead to bone fractures and spinal changes, causing back problems and chronic back pain. Hip or pelvic fractures result in a loss of independence and permanent limping.

Western medicine believes that these symptoms occur because during menopause, the amount of estrogen in the body decreases drastically. With the cessation of fertility, the ovaries cease to function, no longer producing estrogen. The part of the brain responsible for estrogen production fails to adjust to these changes, and continues sending instructions to the body which it cannot obey.

Solutions

The solution proposed by Western medicine is Hormone Replacement Therapy – HRT. The body is supplied with artificial estrogen in order to significantly reduce the dangers and unpleasant side effects of menopause. HRT requires close medical supervision, since it causes side effects (e.g., uterine polyps) in some women. Women with a family history of polyps or cancer need especially close supervision.

In the Far East, menopause is not associated with problems. Research shows that although women from the Far East who emigrate to America do not suffer from menopausal problems, their children who grow up in America and internalize the Western way of life do. Although the tension of modern life no doubt plays a part in this, the researchers' main conclusion is that diet, not genes, affects the existence or nonexistence of menopausal symptoms. Which dietary components are particularly significant?

In 1996, Professor Amnon Brzezinski, director of the Menopause Clinic at Hadassah Hospital - Ein Kerem, Jerusalem, together with Dr. Roger Shaul, researched the effect of soya consumption on women going through menopause. Soya contains phytoestrogen (a natural, plant-derived estrogen) and is a common component of diets in the Far East. The estrogen in the soya bean is absorbed in the body without any side effects, and reduces the symptoms of menopause.

Based on their research, Professor Brzezinski and Dr. Shaul recommend that menopausal women consume soya products five days a week. The range of soya products allows for selection and variation. These include:

Tofu (80 grams a day): Tofu is a cheese-like product made out of soya milk. Of all soya products, it is the easiest to digest and, unlike eggs and meat, does not cause acidity in the body. It can be found in natural food stores and also in some supermarkets. Since tofu is bland, spices such as soy sauce and garlic should be added. When added to various foods, tofu absorbs the taste of the food. Tofu cubes or shredded tofu can be added to salads, soups, boiled vegetables (instead of meat) or desserts. Mashed tofu can be served as a side dish.

♦ **Soya milk** (a cup a day): Soya milk comes in different flavors. Soya milk does not contain lactose and has more calcium than milk.

♦ **Tempe**: Tempe is fermented soya, rich in vitamin B12. It must be

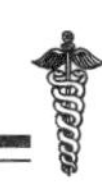

eaten cooked. Tempe can be ground and fried, baked, used to fill veg-etables, made into stew, or added to soups and cholent.

◆**Dry soya flakes:** Soak the flakes for about 20 minutes in boiling water and cook. The large flakes can be breaded and fried, the small flakes can become a goulash, or grinded flakes can be add to ground meat or fish.

Research shows that the following are particularly beneficial:

Miso (one teaspoon a day, five days a week): Miso is a (dark or light) brown spread derived from soya. Miso, like soup powder, adds flavor to cooked food, but is much healthier than soup powder. It contains vitamin B12 and various enzymes. Do not cook with miso. Instead, add the miso to the cooked food (half a teaspoon of miso to half a cup of soup).

Linseed flax (two teaspoons daily, five days a week): Grind the Lin-seed shortly before eating. Leftover linseed should be refrigerated.

Since, according to some naturopaths, soya products slow down the activity of the thyroid gland, algae (seaweed, sea kelp) – which speeds up the activity of the thyroid gland – should be added to a diet containing an abundance of soya products. Some women are allergic to soya products. Firms manufacturing vitamins and herbal medicines have tried to find a solution for this by marketing Genistein, the active ingredient of soya, which does not cause an allergic reaction.

Prevention

Does this mean that we should just sit around and wait for the symp-toms to appear? Of course not! Today it is clear that menopause is a gradual process that lasts a number of years, and its attendant symptoms, rather than occurring suddenly, are cumulative. Prevention is the best remedy.

By using soya products as a natural form of estrogen replacement therapy, you can actually prevent the onset of the unpleasant symptoms as-sociated with menopause. Herbal remedies and physical activity also have a part to play.

Diet

A balanced diet that contains proteins is important. According to the proponents of HRT, a diet lacking calcium can lead to osteoporosis. An un-controlled low-calorie diet to get rid of the extra weight associated with menopause can also be dangerous. Women who wish to diet should select a diet based on the principles of correct nutrition, or consult a dietitian.

Vitamins and minerals

Vitamin C: Vitamin C is a general tonic. It is advisable to eat foods containing vitamin C such as red peppers, citrus fruit, guava (note that guava also causes constipation), green peppers, broccoli, strawberries, papaya, brussel sprouts, melons, and tomatoes.

Vitamin B: Vitamin B acts as a tranquilizer, particularly of the central nervous system. Shoots, brewers' yeast, nuts, almonds, sunflower seeds, and whole-wheat products are good sources of vitamin B.

Vitamin E: Vitamin E helps overcome hot flashes. Foods that contain vitamin E include wheat germ, wheat germ oil, sunflower oil, whole-wheat bread, peanuts, hazelnuts, almonds, and pumpkin seeds.

Calcium+Magnesium: Both help prevent osteoporosis. Calcium is found in leafy green vegetables, broccoli, cabbage, sesame seeds, tehina, soya, nuts, almonds, and milk products. Magnesium can be found in the following foods: bannanas, nuts, seeds, grains such as barley and oats, and cereals such as corn, beans, and soya. Vegetables such as parsley and fennel are also rich in magnesium.

Herbs

Sage and Yarrow contain phytoestrogens. Raspberries strengthen the lining of the uterus. Passiflora is a natural tranquilizer without any side effects. People who suffer from sleep disturbances will find Passiflora helpful. Raspberry tea or capsules and Primrose oil capsules will also help you fall asleep. Lanolin capsules prepared from raspberries or Primrose oil prevent depression.

Physical Activity

In addition to a proper diet and vitamin and herbal supplements, physical activity is essential to keeping yourself in shape. You may also decide to treat yourself to a few reflexology or shiatsu sessions.

Choosing a physical activity is very much an individual matter. It is important to choose an activity that suits you. If you are a yoga fan, be careful since some Hatha yoga poses, such as the candle pose, may be dangerous for women with neck and shoulder problems or with a tendency to osteoporosis. I myself am a strong believer in the Feldenkreis method. The advantages of this method are that the exercises are usually done in a lying position, and therefore are not too strenuous. Walking is another activity that requires only a moderate physical effort. In addition, the average walk-

90

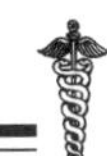

ing pace matches the rate of the body's internal activities, and is therefore extremely effective as a cure for constipation or sleep disturbances (a common feature of menopause). Note that a 20–30 minute walk in the evening or at night is as effective as any slimming diet. It is best to walk on flat ground. (For special exercises see Chapter VII. For preventing osteoporosis, do exercises D 9–10 and D 13–16. For preventing overweight, do exercises A 1–7 and C 10–11).

Walking is not only more fun if you take your husband or daughter along, it also creates a bond between you.

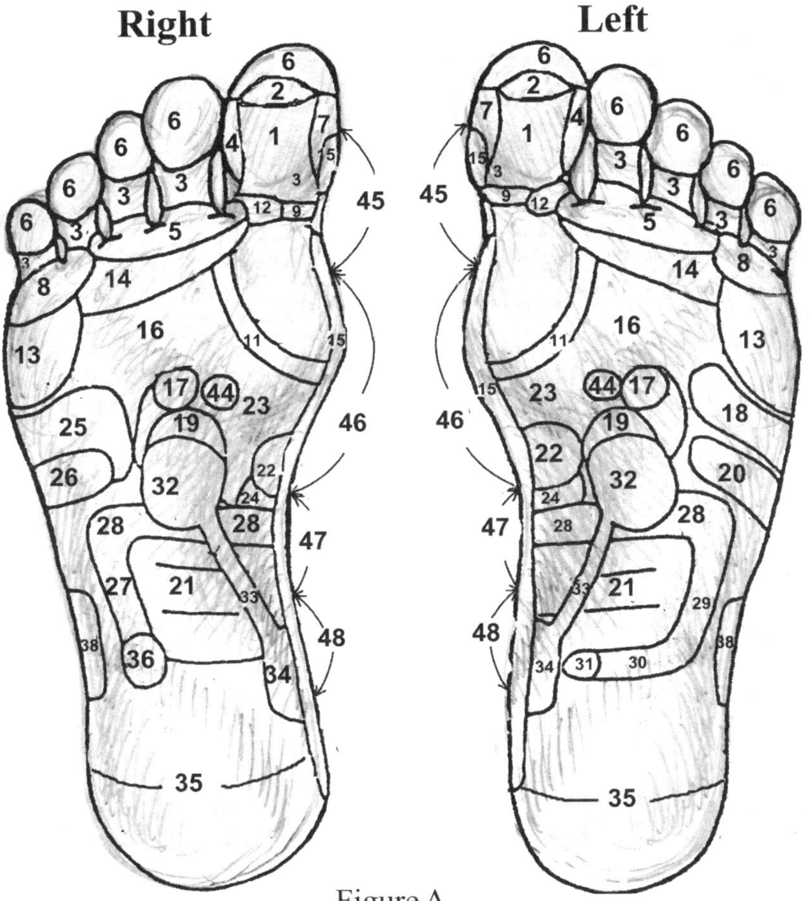

Figure A

Reflexology

After your walk, relax in an armchair and soak your feet in a bowl of

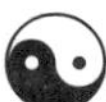

lukewarm water (add a little baking soda to the water to reduce swelling and pain in your feet). Afterward, massage the soles of your feet, using a cream or massage oil as an optional extra. You do not need to be an expert to do this (Figure A).

Shiatsu and Acupressure

Exerting pressure in special areas, at specific points (acupressure) or along certain meridians of the body (shiatsu) can help relieve symptoms, restore the body's balance, and trigger self-healing mechanisms. Pressing along the meridian that crosses the stomach has both a calming effect and a positive gynecological effect. Begin by pressing with your fingers in a straight line from the ribs, down past the navel, to the pubic bone. Exhale as you press.

The following bilateral points are also recommended:

1. **Leg point 1** is good as a general tonic and for preventing surplus weight. It is situated in the soft tissue about four fingerbreadths below the lower edge of the kneecap, about one fingerbreadth away from the outer edge of the tibia (shinbone) (Figure 1).

2. **Leg point 2** is good for hot flashes. It is situated four fingerbreadths below the previous point (Figure 2).

3. **Leg point 3** is the "meeting point of the 3 females." According to Chinese medicine, it is the junction of three "female" energy meridians, and is therefore good for gynecological problems, for the sexual organs, for the elasticity of the vagina, and to prevent painful menstruation before menopause.

This point lies four fingerbreadths above the

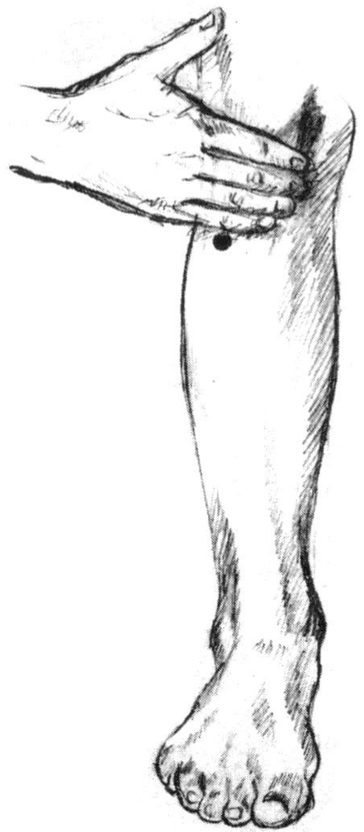

Figure 1

Figure 2

92

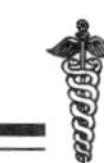

anklebone on the inner side of the foot (Figure 3).

4. The **heart point** strengthens the heart, and alleviates tension and palpitations. The point is situated on the inner side of the wrist, on the fold between the hand and the wrist, opposite the little finger, almost at the end of the wrist (Figure 4).

5. The **lung point** is good for strengthening the lungs and for itchy skin. The point lies at the end of your index finger, about two fingerbreadths away from the fold of the wrist (Figure 5).

6. The **elbow point** lowers blood pressure. It can be found by bending your elbow, until a fold appears. The point lies at the edge of the fold (Figure 6).

These points are the absolute minimum required to achieve the desired results. There are other acupressure points that require professional assistance.

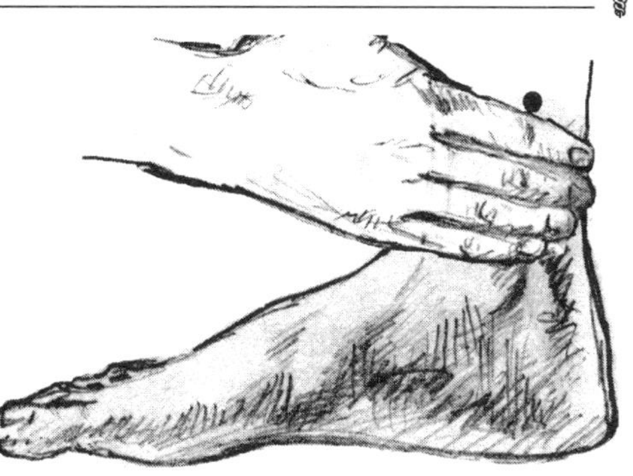

Figure 3

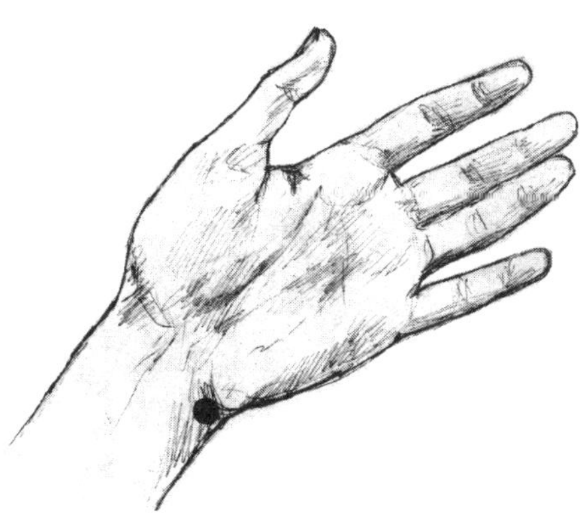

Figure 4

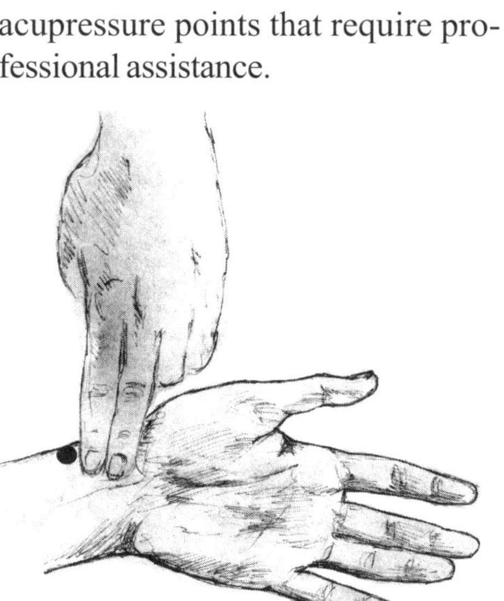

Figure 5

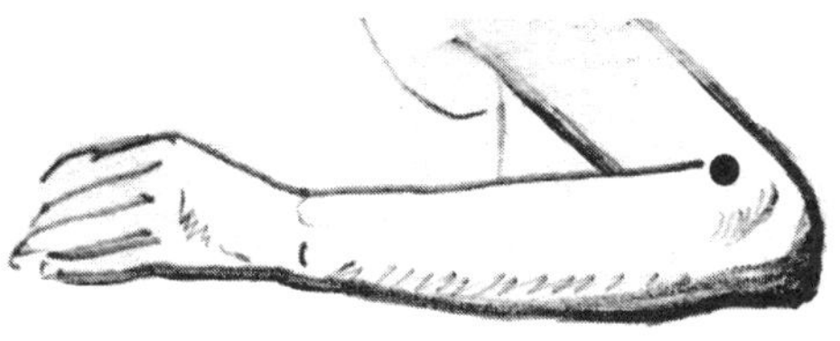

Figure 6

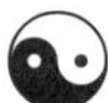

Overweight

Why lose weight?

Losing weight is important not only because a more attractive appearance results in greater self-esteem and psychological wellbeing, but also, and mainly, for your health.

The common misconception that behind those layers of fat lies a 'good' heart is paradoxical, since being overweight damages the body, particularly the heart. Scientific research corroborates this. The excess weight leads to high blood pressure (the "silent killer"), which damages the heart. There's not much point in having a "good heart" if that "good heart" is about to give way at any moment. Every kilo you lose improves the blood's circulation and strengthens the heart by removing fats and toxins and by lowering cholesterol.

According to Chinese medicine (which emphasizes the correct flow of energy through the body), overweight people waste a lot of vital energy on their "overburdened" digestive system, and on "dragging" their surplus weight around. This unnecessary expenditure of energy weakens their physiological and spiritual systems.

One can avoid excess weight by a combination of correct nutrition, a regular, controlled diet, a relaxed way of life, moderate and regular physical activity, a calm family life, satisfying work and hobbies, and a spiritual goal.

Before attacking the problem itself, each person should try to determine why he/she is overweight. Ask yourself some questions.

Is the extra weight due to overeating? If so, why are you overeating? (Are you trying to "stuff" yourself with love? Are you using food as a compensation for deprivation, boredom, or as a cover-up for personal/family tensions, etc.?)

If you overeat because of tension or stress, take Passiflora, which can be obtained as an infusion, tincture, or in capsule form.

If the problem is caused by an accumulation of fluid in the body, drink herbal teas – Parsley, Urtica (Nettle), and Corn Silk.

If the problem is fatigue, pumpkin seeds and alfalfa sprouts are helpful (in plant or capsule form). A mixture of Siberian Ginseng and Ginkgo, which can be found in natural food stores or homeopathic pharmacies, works too. A tincture of Swedish Bitter can also be helpful.

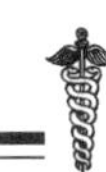

Be aware of your digestive and hormonal systems. Notice how quickly solids and fluids accumulate in the alimentary canal (how often you go to the bathroom). Watch out for swelling in the neck, which could indicate a malfunctioning thyroid gland. If this is the reason, take sea kelp (seaweed), which speeds up the activity of the thyroid gland.

Attack the problem itself by reducing your appetite, speeding up and improving digestion, and finding ways of improving your state of mind and sense of personal satisfaction. Just as "appetite comes with eating" so too, does "appetite decrease with dieting." Chew well and stop eating before you feel full. The Rambam sums this up: "Do not eat until you are full – but stop when you are three-quarters full." (*Hilkhot De'ot*, Chapter III).

Bowel function is very important and can be greatly improved through a controlled diet comprising mainly of vegetables – which is certainly better than using laxatives! Physical exercise, even 20–30 minutes walking each day, helps peristalsis (contractions of the intestines) and therefore digestion. The Chinese exercise devoutly every morning, even on the sidewalks and in parks.

Acupressure, stomach massage in a clockwise direction, and herbal teas (Parsley, Urtica, and Corn Silk) can help eliminate fluids that have accumulated in the body. Dandelion or Plantago, or both, are helpful if you suffer from constipation. (Refer to the section on Constipation)

The following techniques improve digestion:

□ **Reflexology**

Massage your feet. Press the following zones in this order: 23, 21, 36, 27, 28, 29, 30, 31 (Figure A).

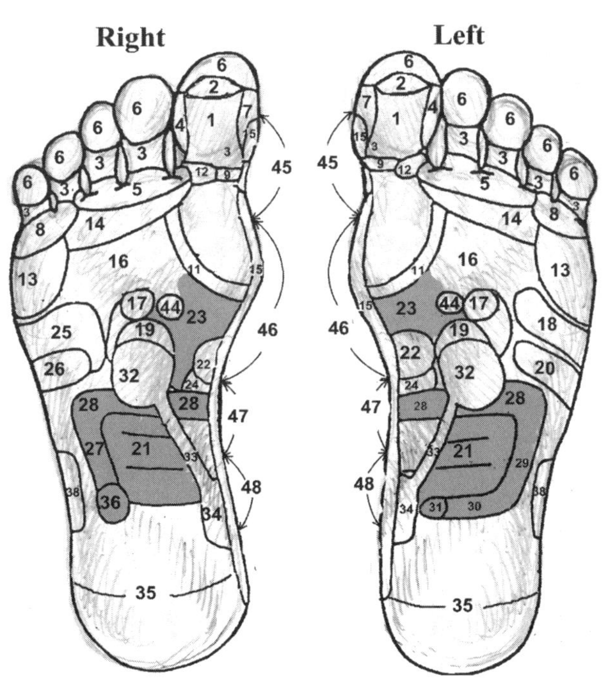

Figure A

These correspond to the stomach, small intestine, and large intestine.

☐Shiatsu

Improve slow or "lazy" peristalsis using shiatsu. As you breathe out, press down with four fingers along the vertical axis of the stomach and the small intestine to just below the navel. Then turn right, and up along the ascending colon, turn left across the stomach above the navel along the transverse colon, and move down along the descending colon toward the left groin. Breathe normally, but the actual pressing should be done as you breathe out through your mouth (Figure B).

☐ Chinese massage

Follow the principle outlined above. Rub the stomach with oil in a large clockwise motion (i.e., in the direction of the alimentary canal) (Figure C).

☐ Exercise

See the list of exercises in Chapter VII. Do exercises A 1–7, C 3–8, C 10–11, D 6–8, and D 9–10.

☐Acupressure

Apply acupressure by pressing down five times, for about five seconds each time, at each of the following three points:

1. The first point is situated in the soft tissue about four fingerbreadths below the lower edge of the kneecap, about one fingerbreadth away from the outer edge of the tibia (shinbone) (Figure 1).

2. The second point is on the outer part

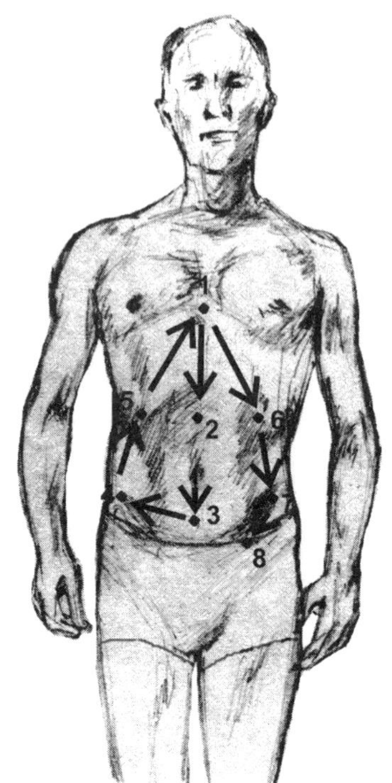

Figure B

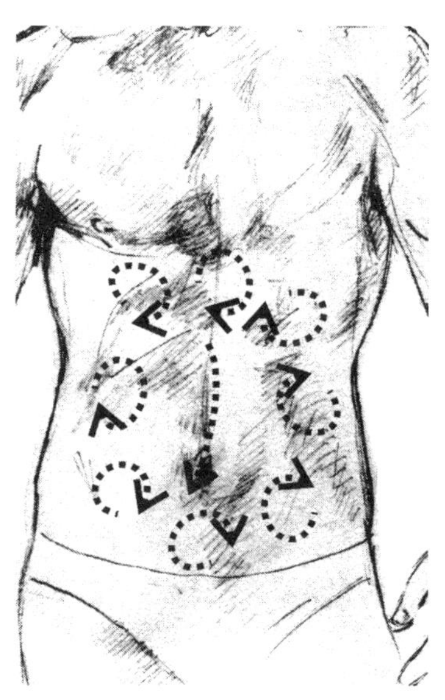

Figure C

96

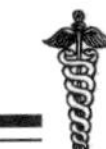

of the arm, about four fingerbreadths away from the wrist (Figure 2).

3. The third point is situated just below your ankle on the inside of your foot (Figure 3). You should keep pressing along your instep, until you reach the edge of your big toe.

Repeat several times at each point on both arms or on both legs.

□ Diet

Choose the diet that suits you and your stomach.

◆ If you can't be bothered with counting calories, do not use a diet based on calories.

◆ If you can't be bothered with a specified meal plan, avoid a diet based on such a plan.

◆ If you can't manage without bread, don't choose a diet that cuts out bread. This would just be counter-productive. You would get irritable … overeat… and put on more weight… Eat 1-2 slices of natural, low-calorie bread.

◆ If you are accustomed to eating a lot, choose a diet based on quality rather than quantity, or a program based on the proper combinations of foods.

In any case, make sure your diet includes all the main nutrients.

Eliminate coffee (causes fluid retention), milk (produces phlegm), sauces and gravies (enhance appetite) from your diet.

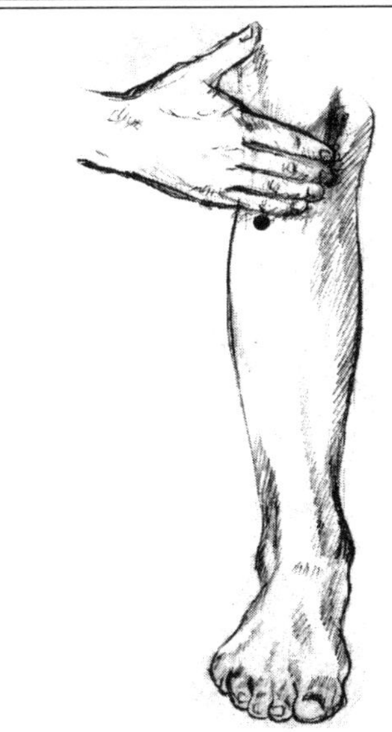

Figure 1

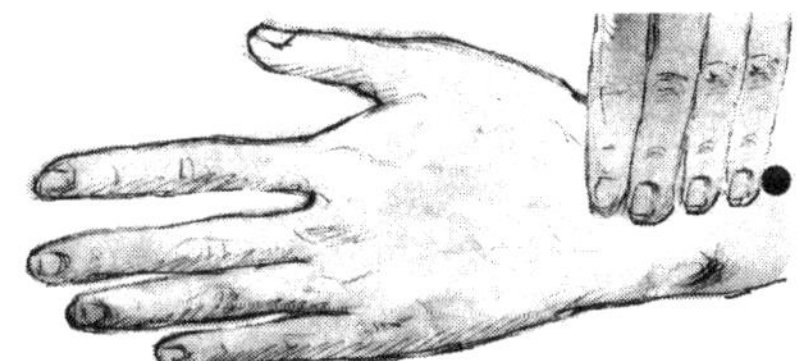

Figure 2

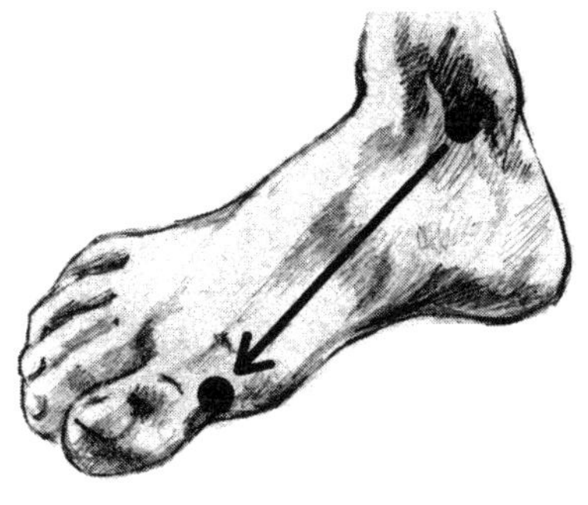

Figure 3

The following table lists substitutes for harmful or fattening foods.

Harmful Foods	Suggested Substitute
Coffee	Bamboo, Hawayij* for coffee
Tea	Herbal teas
Salt	Lemon salt, potassium salt
Sugar	Molasses
Meat	Sea fish, turkey, skinned chicken
Dairy products	Soya milk, tehina, almond milk
White flour	Whole grain flours, cereals, breads, grains

*Yemenite mixture of spices. Different mixtures are used for coffee and soup.

Other useful foods to include in your diet in abundance are:
♦ Vegetables, particularly broccoli, lettuce, and cabbage
♦ Fruit, except for oranges and persimmons.
If suffering excess gas, Carboflor, Chamomile tea, acidophilus, and other natural remedies are helpful.

Good advice: Drink cold water. Cold water forces the body to use calories to warm up the digestive system.

Model diet (optional)
This diet includes proteins and vegetables, but no bread or extras. In order to manage without bread, eat other filling, dry foods. When following this diet, you may have 4–5 meals a day.

Initial stage (2–3 weeks)

The following foods are allowed in unlimited amounts:
♦ Tuna in water, yogurt, low fat white cheese, soya milk, avocado, fish, and eggs.
♦ Vegetables: Raw, steamed, or cooked vegetables, especially green vegetables such as lettuce, celery, broccoli, beetroot leaves, and spinach (the

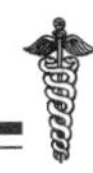

latter contains iodine, also found in fish).

♦ Soups: Vegetable, broccoli, fennel, seaweed (miso), fish, and chicken soups - NOT tomato soup.

♦ Fruit: Apples, pears, grapefruit (between meals), and fruit with a high water content, such as melons and watermelons (not oranges).

♦ Drinks: Herbal teas such as Chamomile and Sage. Urtica, Parsley, and Corn Silk act as diuretics. Dandelion and Plantago have a laxative effect.

Second stage (2–3 weeks)

After the initial stage, add the following foods:

Humus (ground chickpeas) and *tehina* + salad (without bread).

Corncobs, steamed vegetables, vegetable proteins, whole-grain rice, green and yellow beans, *couscous* without meat, burgul with cooked vegetables, green pepper and cucumbers.

Eat food that is rich in essential vitamins. Consult an expert. Prepare filling foods instead of bread. For example, chop up greens, add a little *tehina*, whole-wheat flour mixed with a little water, and herbs to spice. Mix well and bake.

Combinations that provide a complete protein:
♦ Whole-grain rice + green or yellow beans
♦ Potatoes + maize
♦ *Humus* and *tehina*
♦ Soya beans + bulgur or couscous

The diet includes very little oil. If necessary, you may use:

♦ Cold-pressed oil (not date-palm oil) – one spoon a day.

♦ If you want to have oil with your food, add the oil after cooking.

♦ Avocado, peeled almonds soaked in water, or walnuts (not more than five a day).

Walking, exercise, stomach massage, and acupressure (to improve digestion) are strongly recommended.

Sleep Disturbances

*"Sweet is the sleep of the laboring man,
whether he eat little or much, but the satiety of
the rich does not let him to sleep"*.
Ecclesiastes 5:11

The commentaries on this verse explain that laborers always sleep soundly, even if they are hungry, because they are tired from their physical exertion. The rich, on the other hand, have problems sleeping, not only due to lack of physical exercise, but also due to indigestion from overeating and stress. As the Sages say, "The more wealth you attain, the more cares you gain." Thus the Sages indicate two possible reasons for insomnia: indigestion and stress. They recommend physical activity and light meals, especially before going to bed, as ways of combating insomnia.

Proper sleep is vitally important to our health and well being. During sleep, most of our bodily functions work at a reduced rate and our conscious connection with the surrounding world is also reduced. For these two reasons, we usually feel better, or refreshed, after a good night's sleep. Our bodily processes can resume their functioning with fresh vigor. Because we have also had a mental break, we can return to our waking state of consciousness with renewed energy.

Sleep must be truly restful for us to benefit as fully as possible. Unfortunately, not everyone is able to benefit from proper sleep. Many people suffer from one form or another of sleep disturbance. The most commonly used term to describe all forms of sleep disturbances is *insomnia.*

Insomnia can present itself in a variety of ways. The sufferer may experience great difficulty falling asleep, and then, after finally dozing off, will wake up – for some unknown reason – only to experience the same frustrating difficulty falling asleep all over again. Another variation is shallow sleep, where the slightest noise disturbs the sleeper, over and over and over. This poor insomniac never experiences the benefits of deep, restful sleep. In other cases, most often occurring with the elderly, one may sleep well but not long enough, awakening very early in the morning.[1]

Just as insomnia manifests itself in a variety of ways, there is also a

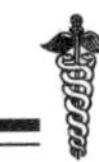

range of possible reasons for its occurrence, and a variety of treatment methods. Many of the differences in diagnosis and treatment result from the perspective from which we view insomnia. From this point on, I will define and suggest remedies from both Western and Eastern perspectives. There are multiple causes and combinations of causes for insomnia, just as there are numerous types or symptoms of insomnia. For this reason, I believe that any treatment for insomnia needs to integrate the various factors and remedies that are available.

Insomnia: Reasons

From a Western perspective, there is a whole range of possible reasons for insomnia:

☐ **Mental tension, emotional problems**

Fear, irritability, and worry can be manifest in a variety of ways, including nightmares and restless sleep. They are the most common causes of sleep disturbances.

☐ **Lifestyle**

Entertainment until late hours, business meetings early and late, political activity, even community service obligations can infringe upon our delicate state of balance and impact our ability to sleep well. The stress that accompanies these activities makes the situation worse.

☐ **Nutrition**

Inappropriate nutrition or excessive food intake, especially late in the day, can cause flatulence and excessive digestive activity that can disturb sleep.

☐ **Irregular sleeping habits**

Sleep is a complex combination of different physical and mental changes. If you go to bed at a different time each day, you upset the establishment of various systems – physiological, biochemical, and psychological – connected with sleep. You may sleep the correct number of hours, but, because the starting time is so variable, the various bodily systems involved in sleep cannot adjust. As a result, the sleep is not restful and you don't feel refreshed.[2]

☐ **Physical problems**

These can include a rise in body temperature, breathing difficulties (sometimes caused by abnormalities of the respiratory tract such as adenoids), poor circulation/cold feet, and poor ventilation. Note: Snoring is not necessarily a sign of deep sleep, but rather of slow, superficial breathing which requires a frequent supply of oxygen.[3]

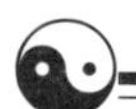

☐ Trauma

Physical or emotional trauma, such as the death of a loved one, or something that triggers the memory of a past trauma that lies buried deep in the psyche or soul and causes the reliving of the symptoms of that trauma.

☐ Side effects of medication

Sleeping pills, antidepressants, etc., particularly when taken before there is a sleeping problem.

☐ Age

Researchers have concluded that after the age of sixty, various individual differences can occur regarding sleep habits. Some people begin to sleep much longer, others for a much shorter period of time. Additionally, some people begin to nap in the afternoon and that affects how long they can sleep at night.[4]

☐ Heredity

There may be a genetic predisposition to sleep difficulties in the form of other health problems, which appear as weakened bodily systems that affect the ability to sleep well. Insomnia, however, is not inherited automatically.

Note: Not everyone needs eight hours of sleep a night. Between five and ten hours of sleep a night are normal. What is important is how one functions during the day.

According to Eastern medicine, insomnia is defined as a continuous lack of sleep, and sensations of fatigue regardless of whether one sleeps well or not. Some people have trouble falling asleep or they awaken during the night. Rather than looking for a specific underlying cause of the problem, the Eastern practitioner examines and treats the patient, not just the problem. By carefully observing the patient's reaction to the treatment, the Eastern practitioner is able to learn more about the patient's condition, gain an understanding of the patient's state of being, and act accordingly. This is of primary importance in Eastern medicine, where everything is interconnected and no symptom exists in isolation.

For example: According to Eastern medicine, symptoms are not caused by only one thing or treated in only one way. A young woman, full of energy and determination, complains of symptoms of sleep disturbances. An older woman also complains of symptoms of sleep disorder, however, she is tired, moves slowly, lacks energy, and her mood is pervaded by sadness. These two women have the same symptoms but totally different "big pictures" or backgrounds. Each would require different treatment.

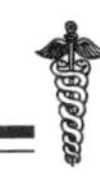

Here are some examples of this concept of interconnectedness as related to insomnia. All of these examples may be connected with stress as the cause, the result, or as a connecting factor, in the difficulties being experienced.

♦ If high blood pressure is the cause, then stress connected with the *liver* is likely to be the source of the problem.

♦ If a sleep disturbance results from fear of an attack of breathlessness, the source of the problem lies in the *lungs*.

♦ Sleep problems caused by digestive difficulties, such as ulcer, heartburn, or stomach pains, are likely to be based on excess heat of the *stomach*, which could be due to stress.

♦ Sleep irregularities due to a ringing in both ears, getting up a number of times to go to the bathroom, or backaches could indicate problems in the *kidneys*, *adrenals*, or *bladder* as their source.

A person needs sufficient sleep. Too much or too little sleep indicates a lack of balance in the body and mind. Insomnia is depicted in many traditional texts as a state in which the person's mind is not at rest. This could be the result of a deficiency of the body fluids (*yin*), which in turn cannot sufficiently nourish the spirit (or mind), which is seated in the heart. In Eastern medicine, the heart is the "home of the spirit" and a troubled heart means a troubled spirit. "The soul is seeking rest" and a good sleep. Excess *yang*, for example, hyperactivity of the body or one of the organs, can also disturb the *shen* or spirit and cause insomnia.

Consequences of Insomnia

In general, cumulative loss of sleep – from whatever cause – is harmful to some degree. Aside from the physical problems caused by lack of sleep, insomnia due to difficulty falling asleep, abbreviated sleep, or situations in which drugs are taken to induce sleep can often result in impaired psychological functioning.[5]

Some researchers claim that the consequences of disturbed sleep are primarily psychological, such as lack of concentration, short-term memory disturbances, and irritability. These symptoms which can lead to nervousness, irritability, poor work performance, and bad temper, can also initiate a vicious cycle where lack of sleep leads to any of the above symptoms which, in turn, can further disrupt appropriate sleep. Worry brings on sleeplessness, which in turn increases sensitivity and irritability, which increases sleeplessness, leaving time for mulling over worries, and so forth, so that psychological impairments may severely affect a person's ability to function.[6]

Physical symptoms can also result from sleep disturbances, including fatigue, general debility, headaches, and burning eyes. Most serious of all, the lack of proper rest over an extended period of time can lead to reduced resistance to illness. Due to lack of rest, the body is not able to produce the nutrients needed by various bodily systems to function properly.

Insomnia: Treatment Options

In the final analysis, there is no one clear reason for, nor one type of, insomnia. For this reason, there is no single cure for insomnia. I will present a number of methods for treatment and prevention of sleep disturbances. I've placed special emphasis on self-help remedies that you can learn to apply yourself by using the instructions and illustrations presented below. Most of these methods involve lifestyle changes, especially in the areas of nutrition and relaxation.

Western Methods

Lifestyle

My father, of blessed memory, used to say, "Don't be awake when others are asleep, and don't sleep when others are awake." By this he meant that a person should keep normal hours. In general, if we have regular hours for sleeping and waking as well as consistency in our daily routine, we should feel refreshed upon waking and energized during the day. However, to achieve this state requires that we become aware of and remove all impositions and distractions. These can include poor nutrition, lack of rest, and negative thoughts such as fear, sadness, anger, etc. To help achieve this state, engage in work that is creative and satisfying to you. Try to avoid distressing situations as much as possible. Return home as early as possible each day to rest, exercise, and devote time to activities you find fulfilling like spiritual goals, hobbies, or visiting with family and friends.

This advice can be particularly helpful for people who sleep only a short time or wake up too early. Instead of forcing themselves to sleep more, they should busy themselves with useful or fulfilling activity during the time they are awake.

If you are disturbed by thoughts or problems that keep you from falling asleep at night, get up and do something. Don't lie in bed struggling.

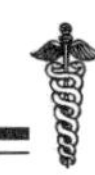

Find something to do that will be pleasant for you and not disturbing to other members of the household.

I do not recommend reading an exciting or scary book before sleeping. Nor is it good to bring your work home and think about it until late at night, especially if it entails excitement or anger. Instead of sitting in front of the television, go outside for a stroll before bedtime. Walking, or a hot foot-bath, can serve as a substitute for artificial devices such as electric blankets.

Relaxation: How to Make Sleep More Effective

Relaxation means the release of tension from the muscles, nerves, and organs, and also the mental/emotional and spiritual processes; it is the opposite of tension. Relaxation is extremely important and most appropriate immediately before sleep. Exercises to induce relaxation can also be useful at all hours of the day.

Relaxation is extremely important for people suffering from pain or various kinds of spastic/nervous conditions. This includes those suffering from irritability, asthma, headaches, migraines, constipation, cramping, disturbances of the liver and bile, stomach pain, and heart pain.

Relaxation Technique[7]

Lie on your back on a firm mattress in a quiet room where you will not be disturbed. The room should be comfortably warm and dimly lit. Remove contact lenses, shoes, and loosen anything that creates pressure, such as collars, shirt cuffs, belts, or jewelry. Close your eyes and gently begin to clear your mind.

1. Place both hands and feet parallel to one another and breath slowly and easily.

2. Begin to think about peacefulness and calm. Tell your muscles and nerves they have permission to relax. Imagine that every organ in your body has become as heavy as lead and is supported completely by the firm mattress beneath you. You can also imagine lying in a warm bath and the soothing water relaxing every muscle.

3. Starting with your toes and feet, relax your muscles entirely. Slowly move up the legs, relaxing the muscles of the ankles, the calves, the knees, and the thighs as you go. Relax the muscles of the pelvis, the stomach, and the chest; at the same time concentrate on relaxing the internal organs in each area of your body, including the intestines and the heart. Loosen the muscles of your upper and lower back, your shoulders, and both the front

and back of your neck.

4. If you wish, slowly turn your head from side to side, keeping your eyes closed. Be sure to do this very gently. Also relax your face including the jaw, mouth, and cheeks.

5. When you have finished relaxing your entire body, rest quietly for a while.

6. Roll onto your right side, then onto your left side, then slowly get up from your bed or mat. Do not jump up suddenly.

7. If you have done this exercise in preparation for going to sleep or resting, there is no need to get out of bed. Simply make yourself comfortable for sleep and drift off.

Suggestions for improved relaxation and sleep

♦ Do not go to sleep too late.

♦ Do not engage in intensive mental activity before bedtime. This heightens the flow of blood to the brain and disturbs sleep.

♦ Think positive. Negative thoughts, worries, and planning are the greatest disturbances to sleep.

♦ Practice breathing exercises.

♦ Warm your feet, especially if you suffer from poor circulation. Use a hot water bottle, a warm bath, or whatever.

♦ Air out the bedroom and then leave the window open a bit, even in winter, so that fresh air (but not wind) circulates throughout the room.

♦ Avoid noise in the bedroom.

♦ Avoid light in the bedroom that will disturb sleep. If darkness bothers you, use a small nightlight.

♦ Practice relaxation techniques like as the one explained above.

♦ Don't try too hard to fall asleep. All the effort geared towards falling asleep only accomplishes the opposite. Merely think about resting, and sleep will come of its own accord. If you have trouble falling asleep, don't worry about it. Relax, read a dull book, count numbers or sheep.[8]

Naps are not recommended for those suffering from insomnia.

An afternoon nap can be helpful for people who are sick, or those with a weak constitution. However, for energetic people or those with a strong constitution, it is not desirable. The Rambam only recommends naps for those who are accustomed to them.

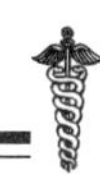

Breathing

It is important to realize that without breathing properly, it is impossible to achieve relaxation, which is vital for useful sleep. Any aerobic activity done on a regular basis will increase your heart rate and improve your general state of health. This can include swimming, brisk walking, running, or other active sports. I especially recommend swimming; it is good for breathing, relaxation, and can lead to better sleep. There are also special diaphragmatic breathing exercises that can be helpful.[9]

Breathing Exercise

1. Slowly and deeply breathe in and then breathe out.

2. As you exhale, expel all the air. Try to extend each exhalation a little longer.

3. Say "sss" or "fff" as you exhale. This will help you focus your effort and expel more air from your lungs.

4. As you inhale, be aware that the air first enters the lower part of the lungs, extending the abdomen and then filling the chest in an upward direction.[10]

There are many more exercises and suggestions. Both popular and scientific literature abound with examples and information if you are interested in pursuing this further. The exercise I have included here will prove beneficial, if practiced regularly.[11]

Herbs

For digestive problems that cause insomnia, I recommend the following herbal teas either individually or as a compound.

Filipendula	**Reduces stomach acidity**
Lavender	**Cleansing effect**
Chamomile	**Cleansing effect**
Aniseed	**Reduces flatulence**
Fennel and Sage	**Soothe stomachaches**

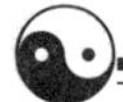

The following mixtures of herbs should be purchased at a homeopathic pharmacy. Tell the pharmacist exactly what you want, as I describe it here, and they will prepare it for you. For these general preparations you will not need a prescription.

For insomnia due to stress, use Melissa, Passiflora, and Valerian. You can use them individually or as a compound. For relaxation, Passiflora is recommended.

Reflexology

Preventive self-help reflexology treatment before sleeping:

Grasp the sole of your left foot. Move it in every direction. Repeat with the right foot. Using your fingertips, massage and exert pressure for a few minutes on each of the following zones: 1,3,6,17,19 (Figure A).

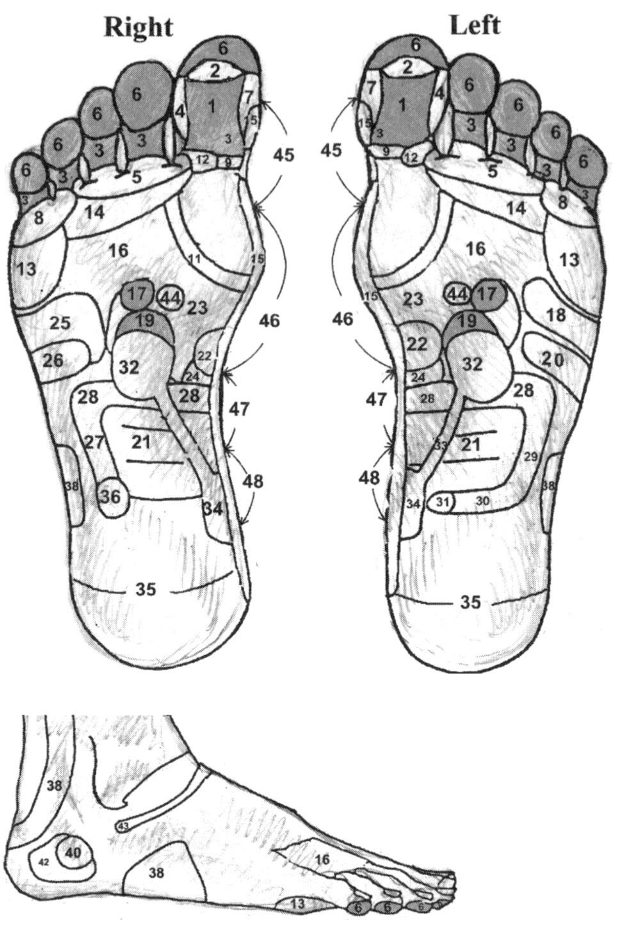

Figure A

Nutrition

The best nutritional advice related to insomnia is to not overeat, especially before going to sleep. A full stomach exerts pressure on the heart and arteries, which causes restlessness and insomnia. If the digestive system is overloaded at night, it will disturb the other bodily systems too. Avoid caffeine, especially in the evening. Do not eat a heavy meal any later than two hours before bedtime, so that you don't overload your stomach. Eat foods that have a relaxing effect, such as a bowl of warm oatmeal, lettuce salad,

108

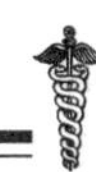

and chamomile tea. See the section on nutrition; the information contained there also applies here.

Aromatherapy

Here are self-help suggestions using aromatherapy for soothing nerves and calming tensions.

♦ Mix with your bath water several drops of essential oil of Neroli or Bergamot individually; or Marjoram, Neroli, and Styrax together.

♦ Massage using oil prepared with a mixture of several drops of the following essential oils: Bergamot, Marjoram, and Neroli.

♦ Tea made of either an infusion or a few drops of essential oil of Bergamot and Styrax, or Neroli alone, in half a wineglass.

Eastern Methods

Lifestyle

In general, the importance of regular daily habits and meal times cannot be emphasized enough. A predictable routine, proper rest, appropriate exercise, and a balanced lifestyle without extremes of either emotion or stress are the optimum.

The Rambam also gives specific instructions to sleep on the left side for the first part of the night and to recline on the right side during the second part of the night. There are both physical as well as psychological/spiritual reasons for this advice. Even if you do not understand all the specific reasons, you can be certain that following this advice will help bring about restful sleep.

There is a Jewish tradition to say a specific set of prayers before retiring at night. In these prayers, *Kriat Shma Al Hamita*, we commit our soul into G-d's care until He returns it to us in the morning. This prayer helps engender a sense of security that our lives will be protected during the night and assured in the morning. Our Sages also say, "Dreams are misleading." Don't put to much stock in them.

Tai Chi

Since problems of sleeplessness are often the result of a lack of proper flow of energy, or stagnation of energy in specific organs, Tai Chi can be very useful in overcoming the problem. The practice of Tai Chi can provide a person with a proper perspective from which to view his emotions. This

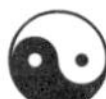

leads to tranquility and a lack of tension, which in turn increases self-esteem, making a valuable contribution to overcoming problems of insomnia. (See Chapter II for more information).

Yoga and Meditation

After many years of personally practicing yoga, I have no doubt that this system is definitely suitable for people who suffer from insomnia, particularly insomnia that is stress-induced. If the physical aspect of yoga is practiced carefully and persistently, a person's thoughts will become calm and his feelings will come under control. The importance of emotional tranquility and evenness of mind for peaceful sleep is indescribable. (See Chapter II for more information).

Acupressure/Shiatsu
For general state of repose:

1. Press three times on the four points on the sides of the front of neck (Figure 1).

2. Press three times on the three points on the back of the neck (Figure 2).

3. Lie with bent legs and press on the nine points of the stomach, in a counterclockwise motion` (Figure 3).

4. Press across the middle of the stomach, points 9–7. Return your hands to point 8, and go to sleep in that position.

For preventing insomnia:

1. General pressure treatment in the center of the temple (Figure 4 - next page).

2. Massage the neck and press on the

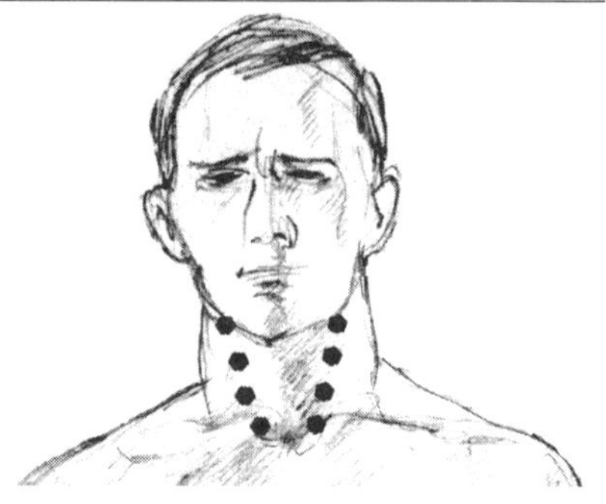

Figure 1

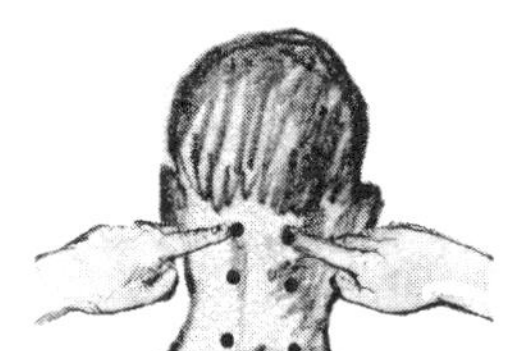

Figure 2

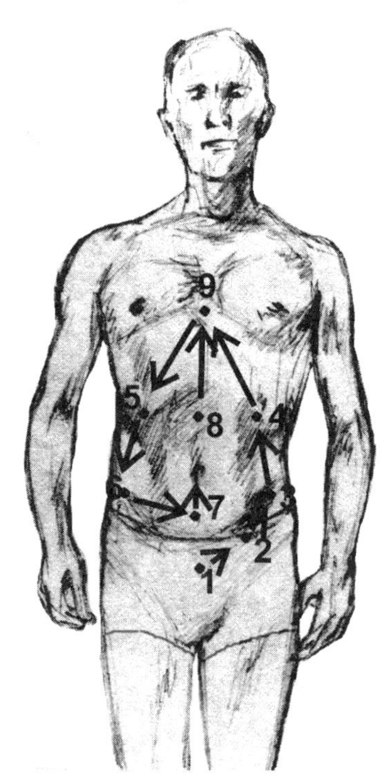

Figure 3

back of the neck, between the third and fourth vertebrae (Figure 5).

3. Give foot shiatsu and pressure on the central area of the sole of the foot (Figure 6).

4. Give stomach shiatsu. This is for general well-being, good digestion, relaxation, and a tranquil state of mind. Sit on your knees and relax your abdomen, or lie on your back with your knees bent and soles of the feet on the floor. Put your hands on your abdomen as pictured (Figure 7a), and inhale. As you exhale, press your hands deeply into the abdomen. You can bend forward to get in deeper. Start this treatment in the stomach area and continue downward toward the pelvic bone, then around the abdomen in a counter-clockwise direction. Do this for about five minutes. You can also place your hands, one on top of the other with your palms over the navel, and rotate in a counter-clockwise direction about sixty times. Then, with one hand still on top of the other, over the navel, vibrate your hands gently moving them in an up and down motion (Figure 7b).

5. Apply pressure to the personality line (Figure 8).

6. Apply pressure to the pain relief point (Figure 9).

7. Apply pressure to the anger point (Figure 10).

As in the case of any kind of treatment, shiatsu is not the whole answer to the problems of insomnia. Even Ohashi, one of the founders of modern-day shiatsu, adds, "Do not take sleeping pills, they make the matter worse. Exercise daily and go for walks.

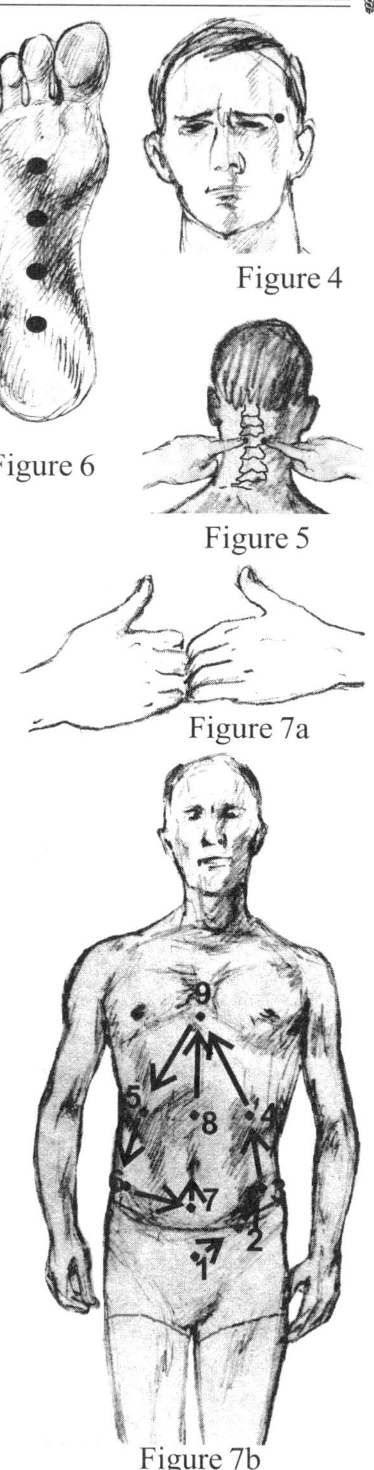

Figure 4

Figure 6

Figure 5

Figure 7a

Figure 7b

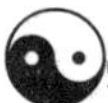

Modify your diet so that it contains alkaline foods, take vitamin B complex. Swim and sunbathe at the ocean; the combination of sea salt and sun are good for repose." [12]

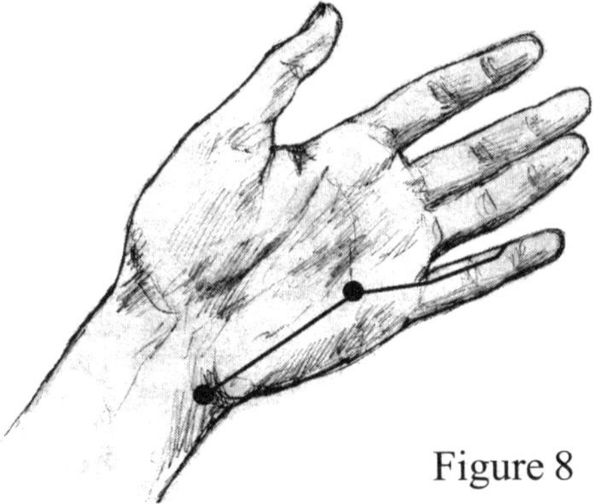

Figure 8

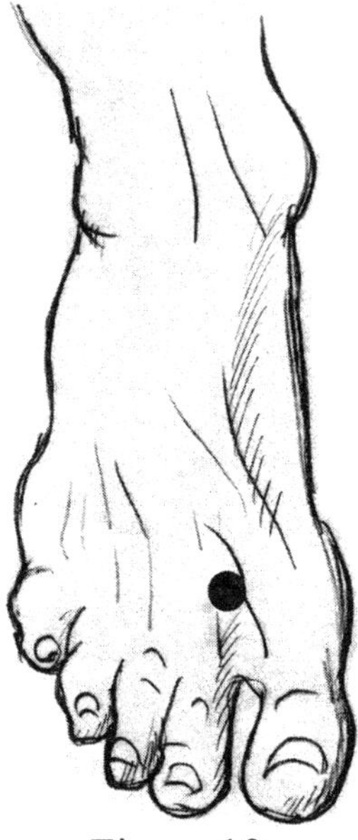

Figure 10

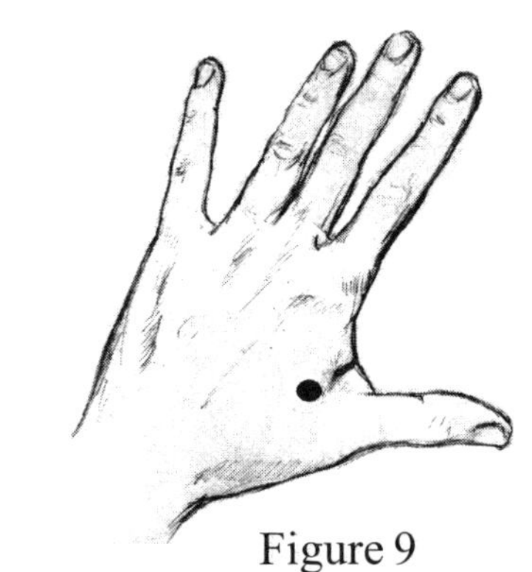

Figure 9

[1] Levin, Yitzchak, pp. 9 - 10

[2] Hel-Or Yom-Tov, pp. 25 - 29

[3] Levin Yitzchak, p. 66

[4] Levin Yitzchak, p.60

[5] Levin Yitzchak, pp. 45 - 50

[6] Hel-Or Yom-Tov, pp. 25 - 31

[7] Hel-Or Yom-Tov, pp. 69 - 71

[8] Hel-Or Yom-Tov, pp. 52 - 53

[9] Hel-Or Yom-Tov, pp. 70 - 71

[10] Hel-Or Yom-Tov, p. 83

[11] Horowitz Ilan, p. 82

[12] Ohashi Wataru, p. 139

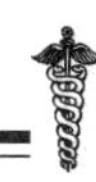

Tinnitus: A Frightening and Irritating Complaint

Do you hear ringing sounds or other noises in your ears? If these sounds start suddenly, at any time, you may suffer from a condition called tinnitus. The pitch of the sounds varies from person to person. Some people hear only **high** tones, some hear only **low** tones, and others hear a combination of the two. Those who suffer from tinnitus complain that the internal noises make life unbearable. Many sufferers try to block out the sounds with earplugs, but the ringing may only get worse. Additional symptoms of tinnitus can include fatigue, difficulty hearing, lower backache, weak knees, extreme irritability, and sleep disturbances.

Tinnitus can be the result of infection, common colds, or allergies. An accumulation of mucus in the region of the ears may trigger the onset of tinnitus. Another recognized cause is damage to the adrenal glands – which sit on the kidneys – as a result of illness, repeated childbirth, or old age.

According to Chinese medicine, the condition is caused by anger or fear resulting from trauma, which causes damage to the liver and kidneys, and ultimately to the spleen. In Chinese thought, anger is associated with the liver and fear with the kidneys. Anger causes the blood and body heat to rise to the head affecting the ears. Fear affects the knees as well. The low-mid back is where the kidneys and adrenal glands are located. As a result, tinnitus is often associated with a weak feeling in the waist and a lower backache.

Excess tension, agitation, or anger are symptoms associated with malfunction of the liver. This differs from the weakness or deficiency associated with malfunction of the kidneys resulting from fear. People with these symptoms usually lack self-esteem and have a great deal of self-directed anger. They may feel so morally and intellectually inferior that they are incapable of holding a normal conversation with anyone. In the event of conflict, they may actually experience a ringing sensation in their ears, thus avoiding contact with others. In such a case, the tinnitus is clearly a hysterical reaction to the conflict. The desire to avoid contact may be so strong that the person finds it hard to hear.

The anxiety and worry associated with tinnitus affect the spleen, which is the seat of intellectual energy (connected to the brain). A weakened spleen can affect the body's immune system. If the kidneys and liver are also affected, the body's entire defense system is in danger of collapsing. In this weakened state a person can easily catch colds, which may affect the lungs and stomach, causing stomachaches and indigestion.

Persistent anger (liver malfunction) can develop into depression. This, in turn, further weakens the kidneys causing a general sense of fatigue. Sleep disturbances are a common by-product of tinnitus. The heightened sensitivity that goes with tinnitus can cause insomnia and nightmares.

According to Chinese medicine, the heart is also affected by tinnitus. The heart is the seat of awareness and the home of man's spirit and soul. At night, the soul usually returns to the heart unless a person is anxious. In such a case, the soul is restless and seeking shelter. When the soul is restless, sleep is elusive. The sleep of a tinnitus sufferer is fitful, interrupted by noises in the ears or nightmares. The patient often wakes up exhausted. Concentration, memory, and other mental and intellectual faculties are affected. Thus, we see that tinnitus can have a snowballing effect, ultimately causing damage to a person's entire system.

Prevention

Although it is difficult to prevent traumas from occurring, and viruses and ear infections are usually beyond our control, as is the aging process to a certain degree (although apparently some people seem to have more control than others, judging by the age they claim to be), there are ways of preventing and treating tinnitus.

A person who leads a fulfilling life will not succumb to trauma or illness easily, and will have the inner resources to cope with whatever challenges come his way. An orderly life, a healthy diet, regular exercise, and relaxation can all help in preventing tinnitus.

Ear infections can be avoided by taking care to dress well in cold weather and to dry your ears well after showering or leaving the swimming pool. If you have sensitive ears, it may be a good idea to use earplugs in the pool.

A well-balanced diet based on plenty of vegetables, fruits, and whole grains can go a long way in maintaining good health and avoiding tinnitus. You should drink enough fluids and the last meal of the day should be a light one.

Remedies

Relieving tinnitus requires strict adherence to the above guidelines, especially the advice about exercise and relaxation. You can also try the following suggestions to obtain relief.

Exercises

Read Chapter VII. Do exercises A 7 and B 3–9.

Reflexology

Press and massage your entire sole and palm, particularly the tops of your toes, the base of your little finger, and the inner sides of your feet, zones 1, 2, 3, 4, 8, 9, and 12 (Figure A).

Shiatsu

♦Lying on your back with your knees bent, use four fingers to press along the line from the bottom of the ribcage until just below the navel, along the midline of the body (Figure B1. See Figure B2 for proper hand position).

♦With your mouth open gently apply pressure on the area in front of the ear, between the ear lobe and the temple. Move your hands to the back of your head and apply pressure on the main depression at the base of the skull with either your thumbs or fingers. Continue applying pressure as you move outwards along the base of the skull towards the depression located under the earlobes. (Figure C.)

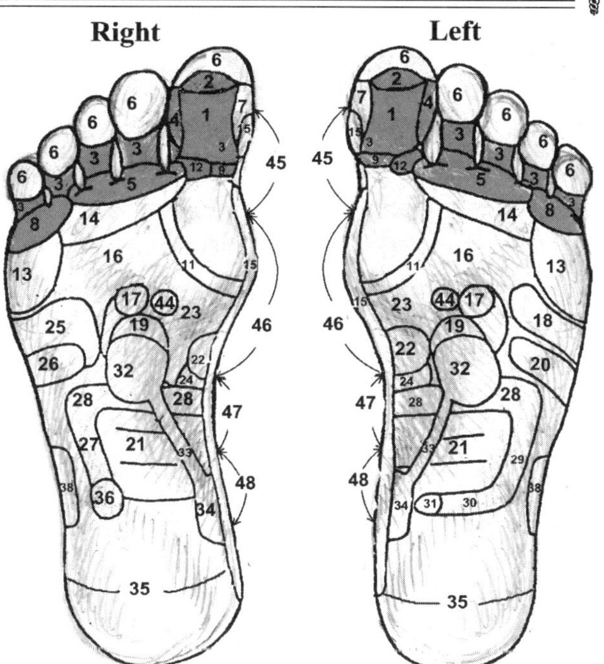

Figure A

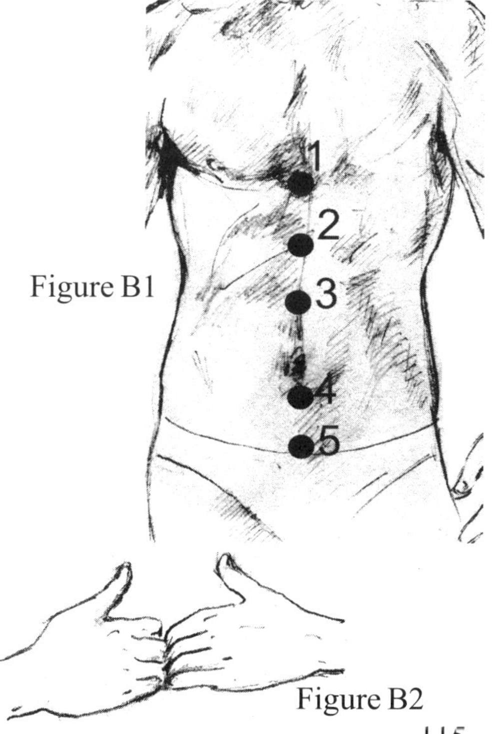

Figure B1

Figure B2

115

Herbs

Both Golden Seal and Black Cohosh are good for tinnitis. Take them either as a tincture, or in capsule form. Golden Seal should be taken to treat fluid in the ear. It is best taken as an infusion. Swedish Bitter, which is also good, is a low-dosage mixture of herbs that strengthens the body. It is taken as a tincture. A pad soaked with essence of Swedish Bitter is effective against earache, when pressed over the affected ear.

Folk medicines

For earaches and infections, heat a little coarse salt in a frying pan, tie the hot salt in a thick cloth, and place this carefully over the affected ear.

Acupressure

The following three acupressure points also provide relief from the side effects of tinnitus, such as dizziness, fatigue, and sleep disturbances.

♦ The first point directly affects the troublesome area. Open your mouth as wide as possible and locate the depression that forms next to the midpoint of your ear. Close your mouth and apply pressure to this point (Figure 1).

♦ The second is a more general point located at the base of the webbing between the thumb and index finger, which works by "remote control." It stimulates the brain to send soothing substances to the affected

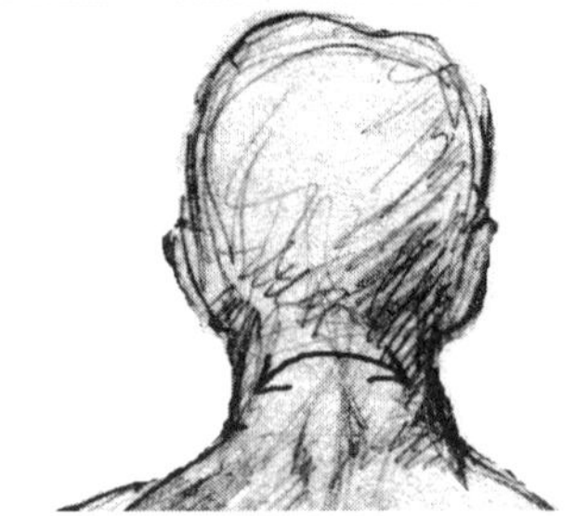

Figure C

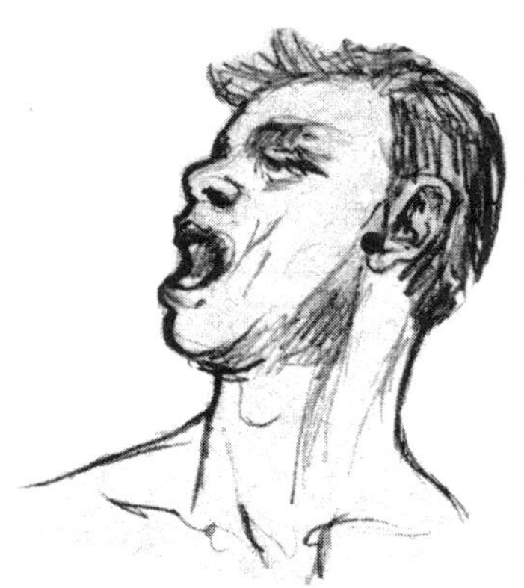

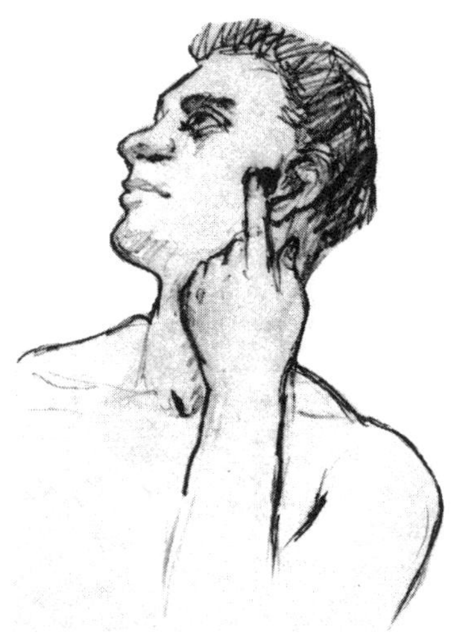

Figure 1

116

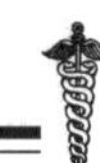

area. Apply pressure gently at first, this point is usually sensitive (Figure 2).

♦ The third point acts on the nerves serving the inner ear. This point is located behind the earlobe, between the mastoid bone and the jawbone (Figure 3).

These additional acupressure points can be useful in treating tinnitus.

♦ Point four is located next to the inner (medial) side of the anklebone, toward the back of the leg. Pressure on this point strengthens the kidneys and adrenal glands (Figure 4).

♦ The fifth point is located on the top of the foot, directly above the ball of the foot in the space between the first two long bones of the foot. This point "draws down" the heat that causes tinnitus and thereby alleviates the symptoms (Figure 5).

♦ Point six is located four fingerbreadths directly below the knee, one fingerbreadth to the outside of the leg bone. Pressure to this energy point strengthens a person. He is then better able to cope with difficulties (Figure 6).

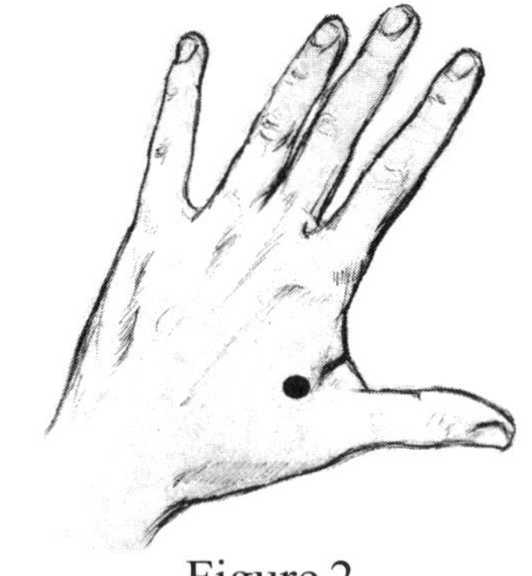

Figure 2

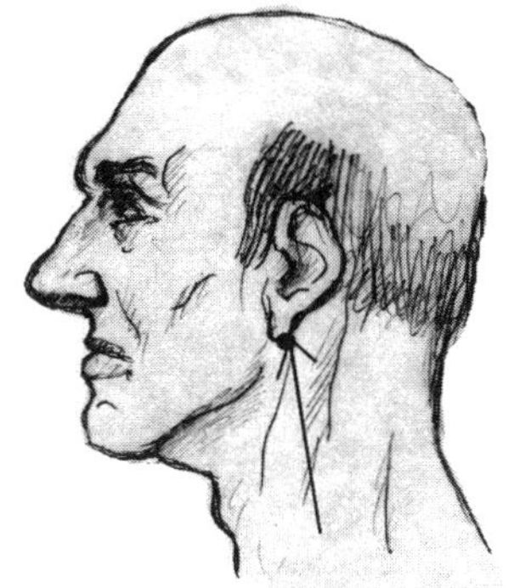

Figure 3

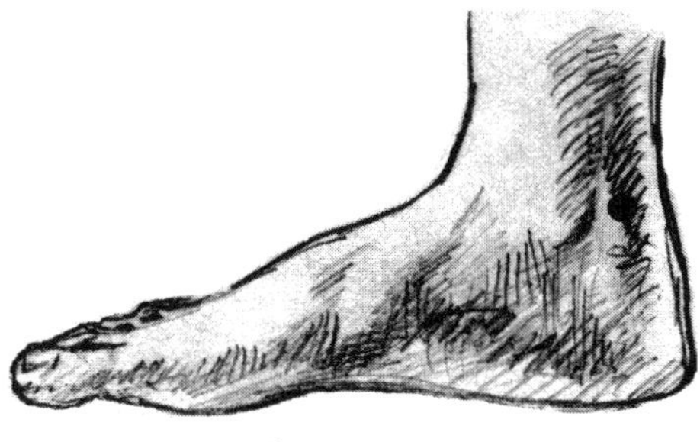

Figure 4

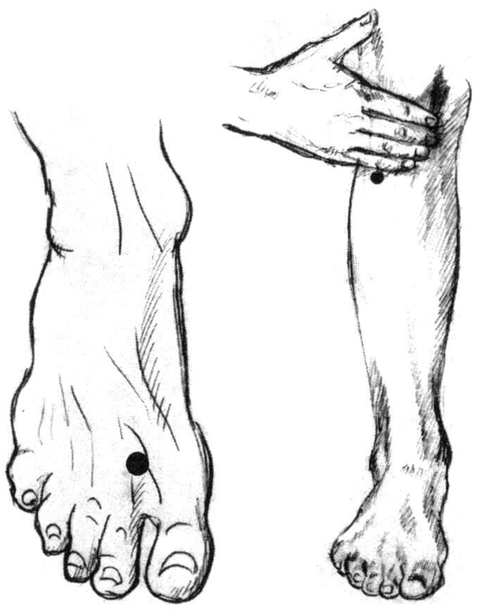

Figure 5   Figure 6

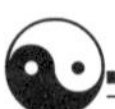

IV. Children's Ailments

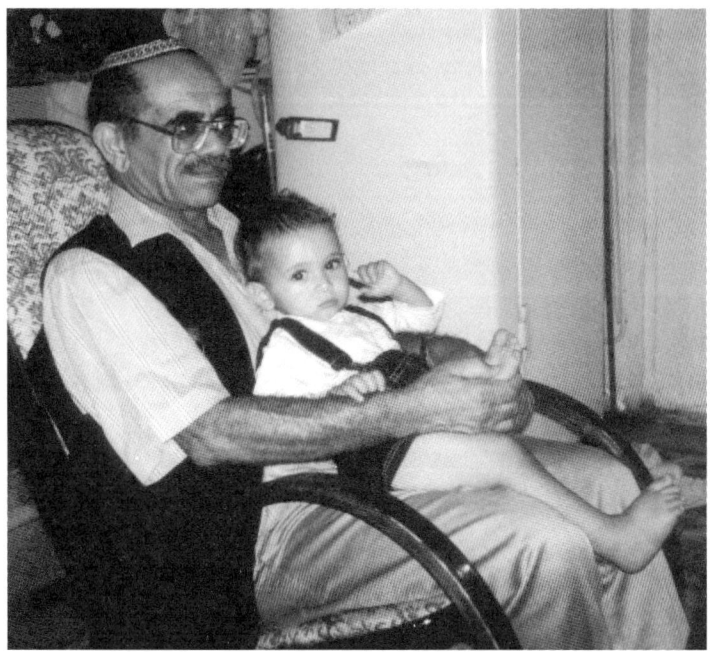

1. The remarks concerning adult ailments are applicable to children's ailments too.

2. Before giving a child an herbal medicine always consult a specialist.

3. Measurements in fingerbreadths referred to in acupressure (shiatsu) are based on the breadth of the child's finger, not the parent's or healer's.

4. Before commencing treatment, familiarize yourselves with the reflexology chart in Chapter I and the map of meridian channels in Chapter II.

5. Figures are numbered separately in each section and not continuously throughout the book (see notes preceding Chapter III).

6. In shiatsu and massage be careful not to hurt the child. Pressure should be exerted up to the threshold of pain, not beyond it.

7. The articles in Chapter III are not intended for adults only. The sections on allergies, backache, headaches, overweight, and others can equally be applied to children.

118

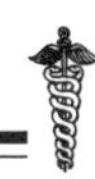

Bedwetting

...It's morning and the bed is wet again... The sheets are tossed into the laundry basket, and the child is subjected to a quick morning shower. A small argument may ensue or simply sad, significant looks may pass between the child's parents, conveying the message that although he's done it again, it's not so terrible. There's still hope!

Western medicine

According to Western Medicine, bedwetting, officially called nocturnal enuresis, is common in children aged four and over, and is defined as involuntary urination during sleep. Bedwetting is considered a problem if it occurs once a week or more, especially if it affects the child, his parents, or the relationship between them. We must differentiate between two types of bedwetters: the chronic bedwetter, and the "recidivist" – a child who has been "dry" for a long period, but has begun wetting his bed again. Usually, this type of problem is more complex.

Often, the parents of the chronic bedwetter never tried to train their child to be dry, for cultural, family, personal, psychological, or philosophical-ideological reasons. As for the recidivist, often a traumatic event causes the child to revert to bedwetting.

Causes

The causes may be divided into physiological problems, family-related problems, parental pressure, and faulty upbringing.

Physiological problems

There are a number of physiological problems that cause bedwetting. These include:

1. Sluggish development of bladder control mechanisms (mostly genetic)

2. Chronic or recurrent inflammation of the bladder

3. A deficiency of minerals such as calcium and zinc

4. General weakness after a serious illness

5. Anatomical defects of the urinary tract, muscular problems in the area, a small bladder, etc.

Family-related problems

A change in the family, such as a serious illness, the death of a relative, or the birth of a sibling, may cause the child to regress. In such a case, bedwetting may be an expression of jealousy of the newborn sibling (he too wants a diaper).

Sometimes, a child is unhappy with his position within the family. This often happens in large families, or with "sandwich" children. The child wants attention from his parents, and when it is not forthcoming, reacts by bedwetting.

Parental pressure

When there is pressure on the child to do well at school and the child does not live up to these expectations, he takes this as a personal failure and begins to feel "worthless." He may try to overcompensate for his failure at school by doing extra well in other fields, or he may regress. Since he equates learning with growing up, and growing up is frightening, he prefers to go back to being small... and wets his bed.

Interestingly, the overcompensation mechanism sometimes has a positive outcome with the child working extremely hard at his studies, usually with excellent results.

Faulty upbringing

Mistakes in the child's upbringing may lead to regressive behavior on the part of the child or to anger, which is then expressed in bedwetting as a way of "getting back" at the parents. The parents, aware of the child's anger, may "pay the child back" by telling him off, or by ignoring him. The child gets even more hurt and angry, leading to a vicious cycle. The tension increases, the bedwetting problem worsens, and the child's relationship with his family deteriorates.

The above is especially true when the child has been subjected too soon to a rigorous program of toilet training. Many parents try to toilet-train their children before they are emotionally or even physically mature. In such cases, the child's behavioral response will choose the path of least resistance, i.e., the urinary system. In such cases, the parents may feel that the child is "bedwetting on purpose."

The above division into causes is purely methodical. Generally speaking, there is no one cause or factor, but a combination of causes and factors. Most commonly, the causes are a combination of the physical (problems

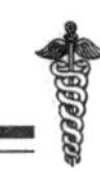

with the urinary system) and psychological (trauma, tension). Sometimes, there are a variety of physical or emotional causes that lead to a physical (psychosomatic) response. Although emotional problems may trigger a variety of psychosomatic responses, when the urinary system is already weak, the most logical response is bedwetting.

Chinese Medicine

Chinese medicine also defines nocturnal enuresis as involuntary urination during sleep and considers it a problem when children aged five or older are chronic bedwetters, or revert to bedwetting. Chinese medicine sees bedwetting as a **condition,** not a disease – a condition in which the urinary system is weak, defective, and cold.

Since the **kidneys** are responsible for manufacturing urine and the **bladder** is responsible for regulating the discharge of urine, the root of the problem must be sought in the kidneys and bladder. The combined weakness of the kidneys, bladder, and the cold factor, affect the bladder's control mechanism.

The above factors may result from a physical tendency with a psychological aspect (lack of confidence on the child's part). Thus, Chinese medicine also sees bedwetting as a combination of physical and psychological factors - a psychosomatic response.

Chinese medicine goes even further and claims that because of the cold factor, the **spleen** is also weakened. When the mind is in overdrive, as is often the case with children who bedwet, the spleen is further weakened (note again the connection between body and psyche), and the child becomes heavy-limbed and tired. This may explain why children who bedwet usually fall into a very deep sleep.

In a nutshell, Chinese medicine ascribes bedwetting to a general weakness of the body's defense system and exposure to colds and various diseases.

Prevention

The Western viewpoint

Increasing our understanding and awareness of the problem and taking care not to exert undue pressure on the child are especially important. Toilet training should be postponed until the child is ready both physically and psychologically. Psychological maturity is as important as physical maturity, especially since there is often a disparity between physical and emotional maturity in children with problems.

If the child still acts like a "baby," crying over every little thing, has temper tantrums, is stubborn, or frequently clashes with his parents and siblings, he is not yet ready for toilet training. Deal with his other problems first and postpone toilet training.

Although I cannot explain all the emotional, psychological, and behavioral aspects of bedwetting in detail, I would like to suggest that you, as parents, consider seeking professional advice before beginning to toilet train your child if you foresee problems. You too may need support. A word of advice: Always avoid confrontations and quarrels before the child goes to sleep. Quarrels tire the child out, so that he goes to bed not only angry but also exhausted – a sure recipe for bedwetting.

Diet and supplements

Proper nutritional habits can help prevent bedwetting. The child should not eat a heavy supper, nor drink a lot after supper.

Calcium and zinc help strengthen the bladder and exist plentifully in the following foods: salmon, pulses (in particular white beans and chickpeas), sesame seeds (tehina), green leafy vegetables, broccoli, molasses, carobs, dried figs, raisins, dates, almonds, hazelnuts, and milk products.

The child should drink enough during the day, particularly herbal teas. Tea warms the urinary tract, and herbs such as Chamomile cleanse it and have a soothing effect on the child.

The Eastern viewpoint

Since there seems to be a correlation between tension and bedwetting, take preventive action before the child begins to bedwet. Adopt the Rambam's golden rule, by being neither too permissive, neglectful, or apathetic, nor too punitive by punishing, insulting, or ignoring the child. Either extreme will not improve the child's self-confidence and will only exacerbate the bedwetting problem. He will feel increasingly anxious, discouraged, and helpless – and a vicious cycle will be established.

Diet

Diet should consist basically of warm food. The child should drink plenty of Cinnamon and Ginger tea, which warm the urinary system and strengthen the kidneys, bladder, and spleen.

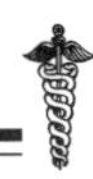

Chinese massage

Chinese massage consists of a series of pulling movements and strokes on the skin that stimulate energy flow in the body. By causing energy to flow along the meridians toward the various organs, Chinese massage creates equilibrium between the organs of the body. It is therefore an excellent form of preventive medicine for all people, particularly for young children. Chinese massage (see exercises below) is also appropriate for of babies only a few months old.

The massage follows the same principles as Chinese acupuncture and acupressure (shiatsu), but massage has the great advantage that it does not frighten the child. On the contrary, it is a source of pleasure and provides a good opportunity for strengthening the bond between parent and child, as the following story illustrates.

A young woman wishing to get rid of her mother-in-law, who was making her life unbearable, went to a Chinese healer and asked for a lethal herb. The healer acceded to her request but advised the woman to administer the medicine in small daily doses and to massage her mother-in-law each day to facilitate the absorption of the poison so that it would look like a natural death. The daughter-in-law followed the wise man's instructions. To her surprise, she found that over time, she began to know, appreciate, and like her mother-in-law. The mother-in-law, for her part, derived tremendous enjoyment from the massages and grew to love her daughter-in-law. The daughter-in-law ran to the healer begging him to give her an antidote to the poison. To her joy and relief, the healer informed her that the herb he had given her was not poison, but simply an herbal tea.....

This story – which many swear actually happened – shows the power of Chinese massage.

As well as being a gentle form of massage, Chinese massage is also very powerful, as the repeated pulling actions penetrate deeper and deeper into the body. When the lower part of the body is cold, massage is a pleasant and effective way of warming the body by causing warm blood to flow freely through the body's arteries and veins.

These Chinese massage exercises help prevent bedwetting. They also contribute to proper physical and emotional development.[1]

1. Support of the spine
Child should be lying face down

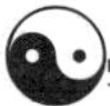

Method:

Use the fingers of your hands and the hands themselves to massage down along either side of the spine. When you reach the tailbone, start massaging the buttocks. Move in an upward direction along either side of the back, "pulling" in the direction of the armpits. Massage in a circular motion around the shoulder blades and then back down along either side of the spine. (1)

Effects:

♦ Strengthens the lungs, heart, liver, spleen, kidneys, and digestive system

♦ Strengthens the back and spine and alleviates back pain

2. Opening the door of life

Child should be lying face down

Method:

Massage the lower back with your palms in a circular motion in a clockwise direction. Take the point above the second vertebra above the buttocks as the center. This is known as the "door of life" and is situated behind the navel.(2)

Effects:

♦ Strengthens the flow of energy in the kidneys

♦ Strengthens the lower back

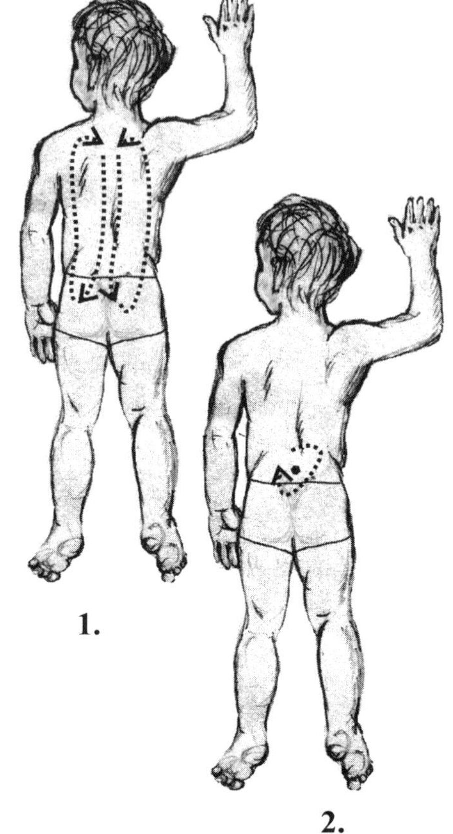

1.

2.

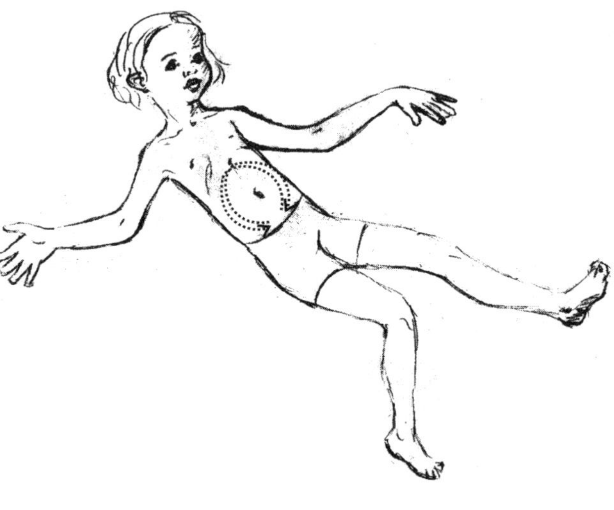

3.

124

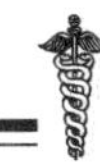

3. Building the fire in the stove

Child should be lying face up

Method:

Massage around the navel, first in a counter-clockwise and then in a clockwise direction.(3)

Effects:
♦ Stimulates the bladder
♦ Strengthens the kidneys

4. Harmonizing fire and water

Child should be lying face up

Method:

Place your hands in the middle of the chest and massage with pulling motions down towards the pubic bone. Move out and up on either side of the body toward the armpits. Massage the chest area with a circular motion, with the hands meeting in the middle of the chest, where you started off. (4)

Effects:
♦ Reinforces physical and psychological stability
♦ Balances the heart and kidneys

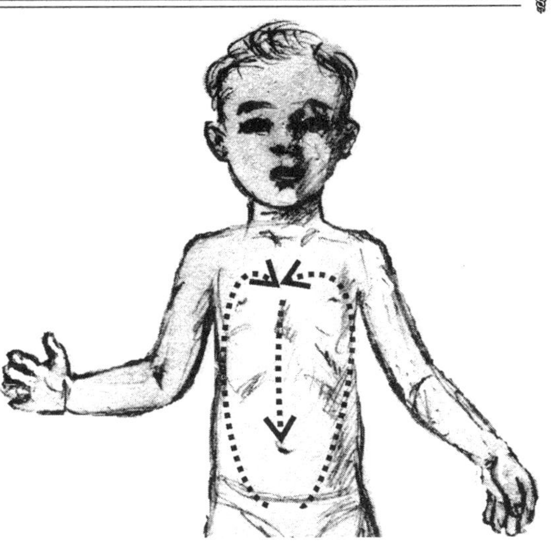

4.

5. Brushing down

Child should be lying face down

Method:

Lightly placing your hands on the shoulder blades, "pull" with your fingertips down the back toward the kidneys where your hands meet. Continue along the back of the legs down to the ankles. (5)

Effects:
♦ Draws heat downward, warms the kidneys

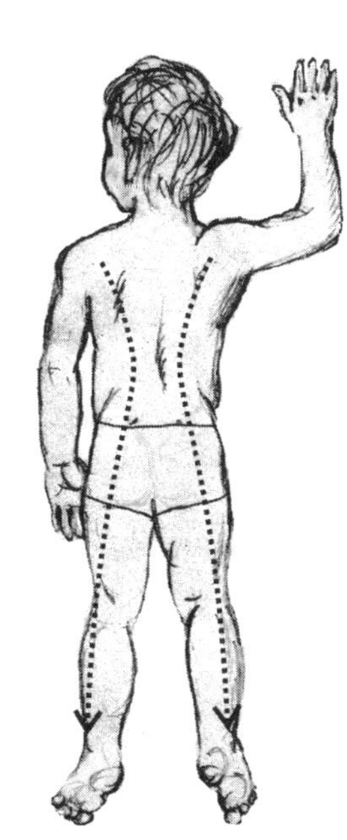

5.

125

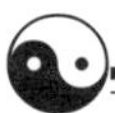

Treatment

The following applies to children who are already four years old and continue to wet their beds or have reverted to bedwetting at least once a week.

General advice

1. Try to reduce tension as much as possible without succumbing to the child's every whim. Always consider whether it's worth getting into a confrontation with the child.

2. Do some thinking. Try to discover the cause of the bedwetting.

3. Find a good time to talk to your child. Try to discover together what the problem is. It could be sibling rivalry; a need for attention, spoiling, and warmth; anger with the parents; a reaction to trauma at home, in school, or elsewhere; the child's sense of being "overwhelmed" or "flooded" by fear or anxiety which makes him "flood" his bed, etc.

4. After you as parents have discussed the matter with the child, among yourselves, and with a specialist; share your conclusions with the child. It is very important to keep the channels of communication open throughout; to help the child understand himself, his problem, and ways of solving it.

Note that psychology on its own is not enough, and practical measures, which may not necessarily be to the child's liking, may also be necessary. These are:

1. ***Cutting down on the child's intake of fluids:*** A popular theory is that the child should not be allowed to drink after 6 p.m., although recently this theory has been challenged.

2. ***The "alarm" device:*** This is a special device attached to the child's pajama bottoms that wake up the child as soon as he begins urinating.

3. ***Taking the child to the bathroom:*** According to this method, the parents wake up the child before the time he supposedly wets, or before they go to bed, take him to the bathroom, and then back to bed. The problem with this method is that it is difficult both for the parents and for the child who resents being woken out of what is usually a deep sleep. Surprisingly, some children do cooperate, although these are usually highly motivated children who are ready to give up bedwetting in any case.

4. ***Teaching the child to "bear the consequences":*** In this method, the child is made to change his sheets, make his bed, put all soiled clothes and sheets in the laundry basket, etc. By transferring responsibility for the problem to him, the mother is "informing" the child that she is not prepared

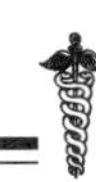

to be the victim of his problem. However, the fairness of this method is questionable. After all, is the child really responsible for what he does? Is he to blame? Is it worth a confrontation and arguments?

5. ***Responding to the child's legitimate demands:*** It is not enough simply to talk to the child and discover the source of the problem. Now that you know what is causing the bedwetting, you have to try and put matters right. Talk openly and honestly. Tell the child that you did not know how he was feeling and that you now want to make amends. Making amends may mean spending more time with the child, being extra careful not to favor other children, etc.

6. ***Positive reinforcement:*** In my experience this is the most successful approach. In this approach, the child is gradually weaned from his bad habit through encouragement, points, prizes, and big rewards if the child stops bedwetting for a long time. Towards the end of the treatment, you should discuss with the child how often he is allowed to wet his bed during the following week. This is a way of turning an unconscious habit into a conscious one so that the child feels he has some control over what he does. Also, by legitimizing the bedwetting you remove the pressure from the child so he is less anxious and therefore less likely to bedwet. (This is like telling a stutterer to stutter – he often ends up speaking fluently).

As the child improves, praise his efforts and show him you believe he can overcome the problem. If he says he wants to stop bedwetting, believe him! Most children do not wish to continue a habit that causes them suffering. Children who bedwet cannot sleep over at friends, relatives, on trips, or sleepover camp. Older children may worry that their clothes smell of urine. Bedwetting is a habit they can do without!

Be careful not to overdo the verbal encouragement and praise. You may, however, sometimes decide to "overlook" a relapse, or give the child a small prize even if he "doesn't really deserve it."

In addition to emotional–psychological reinforcement, the child will benefit from physical remedies such as a proper diet, supplements, and herbs.

Diet and supplements

The dietary advice specified under "preventive measures" above may also be applied to treating bedwetting. In addition, children with weak bladders should refrain from eating white sugar or sweets. Sugar "destroys" the body's calcium – already in short supply – making the bladder even weaker.

As alternatives to "sweets" give your children fruit or sweets made with carob, honey, molasses, etc. Almonds, hazelnuts, dried figs, raisins, and dates also serve as healthy alternatives to candies in addition to being rich in calcium and zinc.

Give your child vitamin C by serving him fruit and vegetables rich in vitamin C, such as citrus fruit, kiwi, guava, green pepper, broccoli, strawberries, papaya, brussels sprouts, and tomatoes.

Herbs

The following formula, 30 drops in water, three times a day, is recommended.

Mix equal amounts of:

Passiflora – tranquilizing agent

Uva Ursi (Blueberries) – for urinary tract infections

Echinacea(Cone Flower) – for strengthening the immune system

Urtica (Nettles) – for urinary tract problems

Alfalfa (Lucerne) – a general tonic.

This can also be taken as a tea.

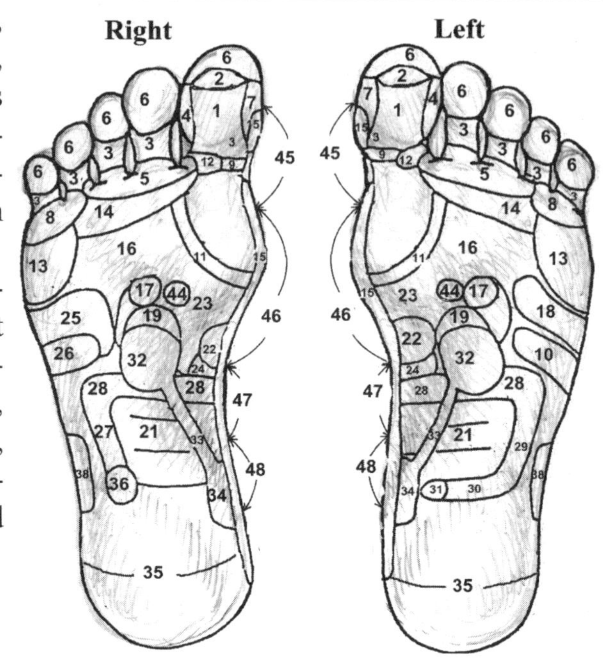

Figure A

Additional remedies

☐**Rest** during the day.

☐**Chinese massage**, or any massage, is usually enjoyed by the child.

☐**Acupuncture and acupressure**

Although acupuncture is effective, many children are afraid of it. Therefore, **reflexology** (massage of the sole), **shiatsu** (finger pressure along specific lines), and **acupressure** (pressing specific spots) are the preferred treatments.

☐**Reflexology**

Reflexology consists of massaging and kneading the entire area of the

128

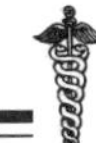

sole. This helps relax and strengthen the entire body (Figure A).

☐Shiatsu

1. Press down on either side of the neck, about a fingerbreadth away from the first vertebra, from the base of the head along to the shoulders.

Continue pressing down on the spinal muscles, two fingerbreadths away from the spine, down to the hips and tailbone. This line contains points that connect with all body organs, depending on their location in the body. Acupressure along this line relaxes tense muscles, straightens the spine, and strengthens the body (Figure B1).

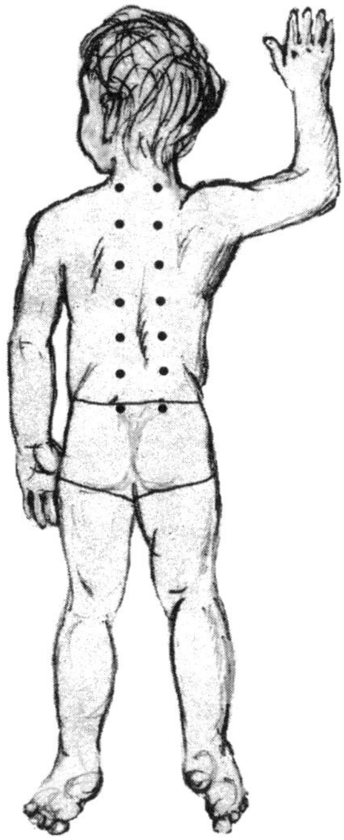

2. Press down with the fingers of both hands on either side of the sacrum, tailbone, and buttocks, about two fingerbreadths from the spine. Press with both thumbs on every point from top to bottom (Figure B2).

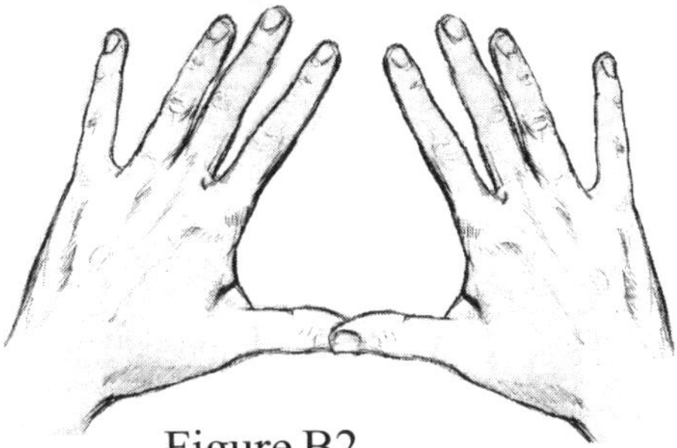

Acupressure points

1. Neck point: This point is situated about a fingerbreadth away from the spine, on either side, along the natural hairline (Figure 1).

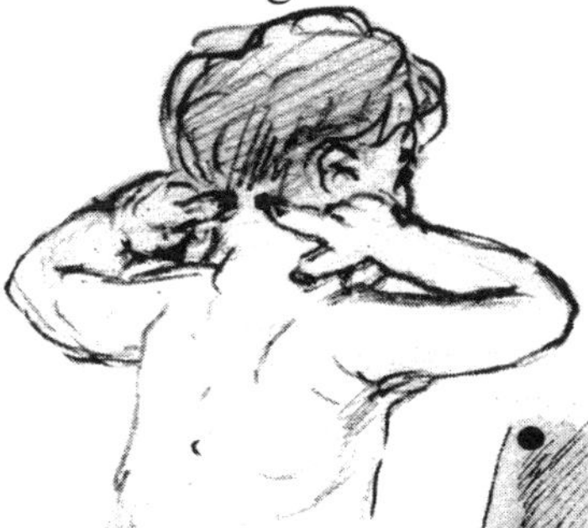

2. Foot point: This point forms the junction of three energy lines: liver, spleen, and kidney. It is situated about four fingerbreadths above the anklebone on the inner side of the leg (Figure 2).

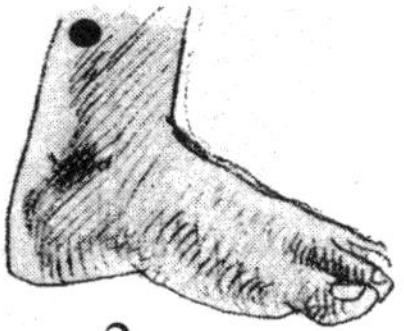

Figure B1

Figure B2

Figure 1

Figure 2

3. ***Lower stomach point***: This point is situated about six fingerbreadths below the navel and serves as the bladder's "warning point." It strengthens the lower part of the body, especially the bladder (Figure 3).

4. ***Head point***: Acupressure at this point lightens the heavy sleep that is characteristic of children who bedwet. Draw an imaginary line from the ears to the top of the head, and from the nose to the top of the head. The head point is located at the junction of these lines. You can either press on this point or tap it with your knuckles (Figure 4).

5. ***Hand point***: This point has a tranquilizing and relaxing effect. It is situated on the inner fold of the wrist, opposite the little finger (Figure 5).

6. ***Ankle point***: Acupressure at this point strengthens the energy of the kidneys and the bladder. It is situated between the ankle and the Achilles tendon, in the dimple behind the inner anklebone (Figure 6).

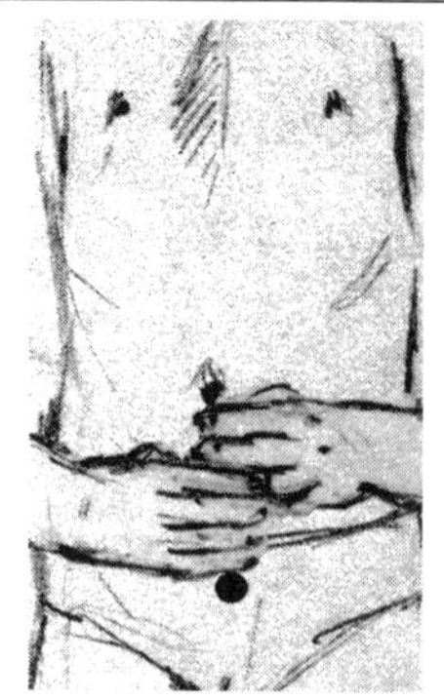

Figure 3

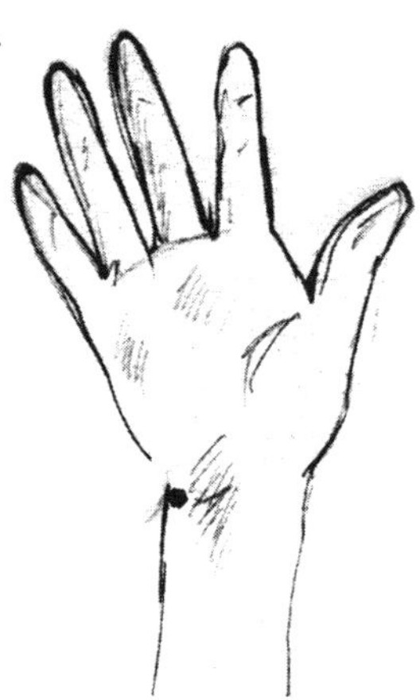

Figure 5

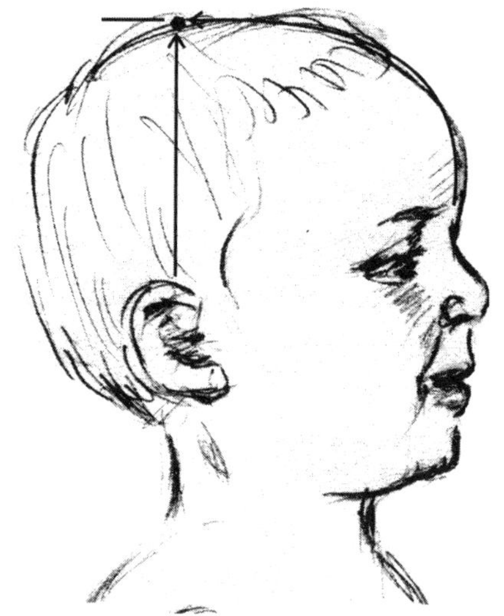

Figure 4

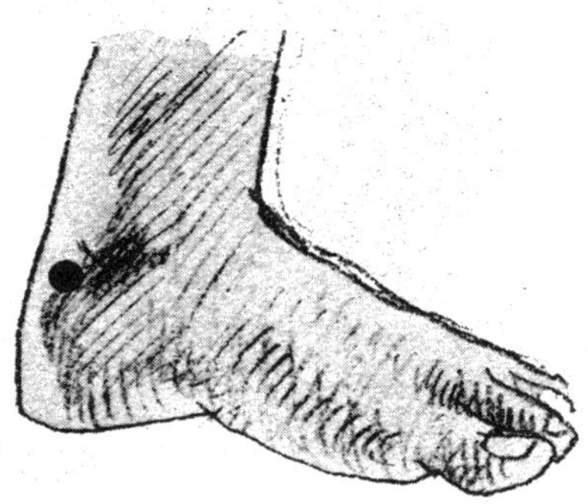

Figure 6

[1]Russell and Gordon, pp. 16–17, 20–23, 32–33, 38–39, 76–77.

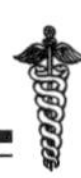

Children's Colds

I was once asked the following question: What can be done to prevent recurrent colds in children? Let me begin by saying that the advice I gave in "The Common Cold" also applies to children, although some common sense is required in applying the advice to children.

What is meant by common sense? Let us take fever as an example. Although fever is one of the body's ways of fighting illness, a temperature of over 39 degrees Centigrade can be dangerous for children. A high fever may even induce convulsions in some children, causing irreversible brain damage. Although the child may recover, he may be left with physical developmental problems, and learning and social difficulties.

I cannot stress how wrong it is when parents assert their moral right over their children's health and refuse active medical intervention when there is a vital need for it. I know of a number of cases where the parents' lack of flexibility damaged their children's health. On the other hand, parents cannot always be blamed, since often everything seems normal on the surface. A child with a high temperature may seem to be happy and in good spirits (sometimes too much so, and if he/she is delirious, the child may even speak nonsense). However, a sudden switch from energy to lassitude, when the child suddenly goes limp "like a rag," should serve as a warning signal that something is not right, and action should be taken immediately. Therefore, if a child has a fever of over 39 degrees Centigrade, immediate steps must be taken to lower the temperature.

Some mothers believe it is good to expose a child with a high fever to wind and cold claiming that the "child has to develop immunity." Chinese and Eastern medicine strictly forbids exposure to cold or wind. Wind, in Eastern medicine, is considered one of the main causes of illness. What Western medicine calls a "virus" or "bacteria" – Eastern medicine defines as the body succumbing to an attack of wind, cold, or heat due to a weakened body system. Therefore, Eastern medicine concludes that one has to adapt one's diet and clothes to the weather. In the winter, for example, you should dress more warmly, eat hotter foods, and be more careful when moving from a warm to a cold environment. We are familiar with the Rambam's advice that one should not leave a bathhouse immediately, but rather one should protect himself from the wind by warming up in the lobby before going out.

The above is even more true for children, since their immune system is not yet completely developed. The immune system comprises the lungs, skin, body hair, and nasal passages. The external pathogenic element, whether "wind" in Chinese thinking, or a "virus" in Western thinking, can penetrate the body via the nose, mouth, or skin. This explains why the symptoms of a cold take the form of cold and heat, shivering and perspiration, sneezing, runny nose, and coughing.

Prevention

1. General: Your best bet is to follow the Rambam's "golden mean." You don't have to wrap your child in five sweaters, but neither should you allow him to go wet from the shower to his room when there is a strong draft. You must take into account both the weather and the child's physical condition.

2. Protect your child: The room in which your child sleeps should be well ventilated but should not have a northern or western exposure. If the window has a northern or western exposure, you should close the window and leave the door open.

3. Diet: Weak children can regain their strength through a proper diet. Healthy food also has an antibiotic effect and strengthens the body. The child should eat plenty of fruit, vegetables, and whole grains. Try to avoid foods that contain white flour, white sugar, etc.

4. Vitamins: Give your child vitamin C daily throughout the winter. Because vitamin C tablets can cause diarrhea, serve foods that have plenty of vitamin C such as broccoli, guava, red peppers, melon, citrus fruit, kiwi, strawberries, etc. Rose Hips syrup is an excellent source of vitamin C without any side effects.

5. Herbs: Some herbs act as antibiotics and also strengthen the body's immune system, unlike ordinary antibiotics which weaken the body's natural resistance. However, in cases of serious infections or inflammations, parents should follow the instructions of their conventional doctor.

To strengthen the immune system, try the following as a tincture:
1. Echinacea – strengthens the immune system
2. Propolis — antibiotic
3. Equisetum – anti-allergen
4. Chamomile – anti-inflammatory

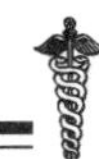

Depending on the age of the child and the instructions of the homeopathic pharmacist, mix several drops of the formula with a little water and let the child drink it three times a day on an empty stomach. The formula or part of it can also be taken as a syrup or tea. Continue this as long as necessary.

Between bouts pay attention to the following:

The psychological aspect

The child may be experiencing social or other problems at the day care center, nursery school, or primary school. Alternatively, the child might like being at home and getting attention. He or she may also be jealous of a new brother or sister. When the child is "ill" he/she is able to "watch over" the mother and make sure she does not devote herself to the new baby.

I know of a child who, when he made up his mind not to go to school, would wake up the next day with a temperature of 39 degrees Centigrade.

The physiological aspect

You must make sure that the child is not suffering from a food or other allergy.

Allergies can cause cold-like symptoms. The body's immune system may interpret pollen and dust as an external attack and may respond to certain foods as an internal attack. Allergies are a case of mistaken diagnosis by the body. The body's "intelligence system" sees shadows as the "enemy," and then recruits all its ammunition (sneezing, runny nose, tearing eyes, temperature, etc.) to fight the "enemy." The symptoms may mimic all the symptoms of a cold or flu. After the body has been weakened from this "tilting at windmills," a real cold or flu may actually develop, triggered by an internal or external cause. Therefore, in cases of recurrent colds, a process of elimination should be used to determine what the child might be allergic to. This may be done by a natural healer or in a laboratory that specializes in allergies.

Various herbs can alleviate allergic reactions. The following herbs can be taken individually or in combination, as advised by an herbal specialist.

◆ Equisetum – anti-allergen.

◆ Liquorice – an effective expectorant that helps alleviate coughing spasms.

♦ Astragalus – a Chinese herb that strengthens the immune system.

♦ Feverfew – for flu-associated headaches. This should be continued even after the headache has disappeared as a preventive measure.

♦ Pollen extract – strengthens the body.

♦ Sambucus (Elder) – a plant that is effective against viruses of all kinds, especially flu and coughs. It can be added to the formula or taken separately (in syrup form). It can be used as a preventive or as a curative agent.

Treatment

As a treatment, all the above advice should be applied more intensively.

1. ***Caring for a sick child:*** Children sometimes enjoy being ill because they get extra attention. While it is important to give legitimacy to their feelings, be careful not to pamper them too much, or feel to sorry for them. Once again one should follow the golden mean. One should neither show too much anxiety, nor accuse the child of being "spoiled" or "seeking too much attention."

2. ***Diet and rest:*** Fasting can actually help a child recover. In any case, sick children usually do not have much of an appetite. This is nature's way of ensuring that the body does not "waste" energy digesting food, but uses it to recuperate. Sick children need lots of rest to allow the body to fight the disease. The problem with children, however, is that we cannot always get them to do what we want. It is amazing how children's reactions differ. Some children with fever will run around the house or jump on mattresses, while other will lie quietly in bed even when they do not have a fever. This may be because children with lots of energy (Yang, in Chinese medicine) have a stronger and faster reaction to illness and recover more quickly. While those with a weaker constitution (Yin, in Chinese medicine), take longer to recover and are more likely to suffer repeated bouts of illness. Active children should not be allowed to run around too much, but should be kept occupied in bed.

3. ***Lowering fever:*** When a child has a high temperature it must be lowered. This can be accomplished by wiping the child's forehead, chest, stomach, and back with a wad of cotton wool soaked in water. Do this repeatedly while the temperature is rising. If there is a danger of convulsions, the child should be placed in a tub of lukewarm water or in a shower. If the fever rises again soon after, consult a doctor immediately. Give the child plenty to drink in order to compensate for the loss of body fluids caused by

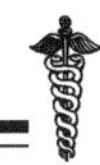

the fever. It is best to give lukewarm drinks, not hot ones, since a hot drink raises the body's temperature. A lukewarm drink lowers the body's temperature by helping the child perspire. The best drinks are herbal teas such as Chamomile, Cinnamon, Eucalyptus leaves, Mint, Sage, and Cloves.

A child who has already stopped using a bottle may insist on drinking with a bottle when sick. It might be wise to let him have his way since the important thing here is for him to drink. Hopefully, he won't get too used to it.

The child will want to throw off his blankets, especially if he has high fever. However it is important to prevent him doing this. Covering and keeping the child warm helps the child perspire which lowers his temperature.

4. ***Treating catarrh (a nasal cold):*** Use a warm humidifier with eucalyptus oil added. If the child does not respond well, or you don't have a humidifier, hang wet towels around the room, on the radiators and on every available spot. The humidity also helps sore throats and coughs. According to Chinese medicine, humidity helps strengthen weak lungs. (Note: If you use a cold humidifier, Eucalyptus oil should not be added).

5. ***Treating coughs:*** The following home-made remedies are helpful:

♦ At night, before going to sleep, rub olive oil on your child's chest. Sprinkle coarse salt over the oil and spread a thin piece of nylon sheeting or newspaper over it. The child should then put on a warm undershirt. This remedy is extremely effective against coughs, mucus, and phlegm.

♦ Mix lemon juice and honey in equal amounts and give the child two teaspoons three times a day.

♦ For small children and toddlers: Dip a slice of bread in olive oil and feed the child bit by bit. This remedy helps break down phlegm and relieves coughs.

6. ***Persistent coughing with danger of pneumonia:*** Windcupping is an effective remedy against pneumonia. Cups placed on the skin create a vacuum, increasing the flow of blood in that area. Before antibiotics were invented, my grandmother and mother used windcupping to save the lives of hundreds of children who were dangerously ill with pneumonia. Today, this "old-fashioned" remedy is being used more and more. There are healers who specialize in windcupping.

7. ***Stomachaches:*** If your child has a stomachache, begin by massaging the soles of his feet. Once the stomachache is less acute, gently massage olive oil into the stomach. Be aware that a sharp pain on the right side may be appendicitis.

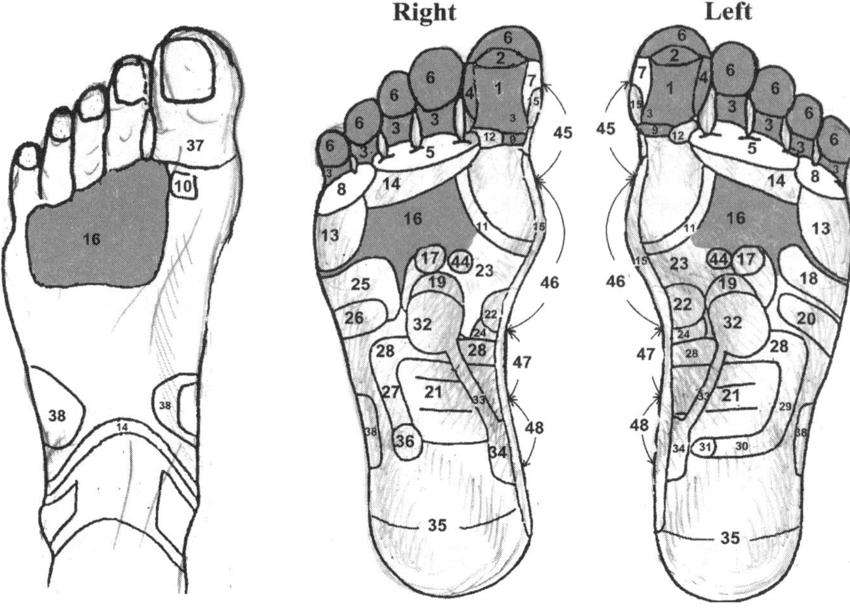

Figure A

8. *Earache:* Heat a little cooking salt in a dry frying pan, pour into a cloth, and carefully place over the affected ear. Hopefully, the salt will draw out the fluid in the ear and alleviate the pain.

Reflexology

Give the feet a general massage, and then concentrate on zones 1, 2, 3, 4, 6, 9, and 16 (Figure A).

Acupressure

Fingerbreadth refers to the child's fingers.

♦ *For blocked nose or catarrh:* Press the spots adjacent to the nostrils on either side of your nose. Other points are the middle

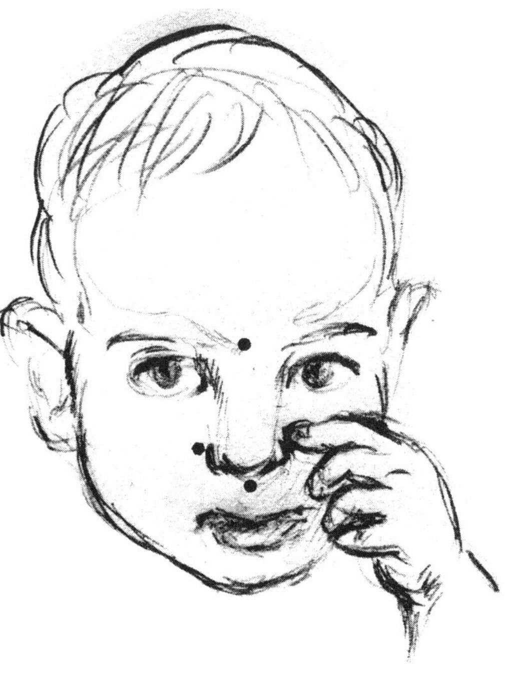

Figure 1

136

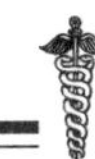

of the upper lip and between the eyebrows (Figure 1).

♦ *For sore throats and general aches and pains*: The point is located on the back of your hand, just below the mound formed by the junction of thumb and index finger, between the two bones. With your thumb, press down, inward (Figure 2).

♦ *For coughs and breathing problems*: The point lies two fingerbreadths away from the fold of the wrist, on the inner side of the wrist (Figure 3).

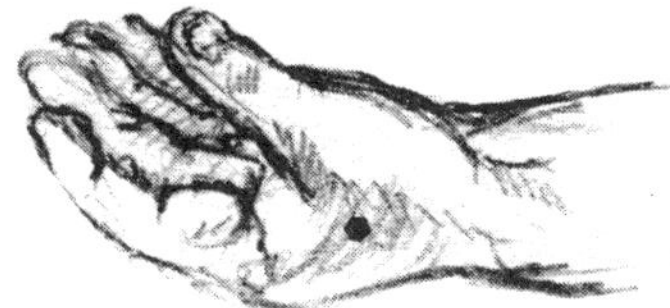

Figure 2

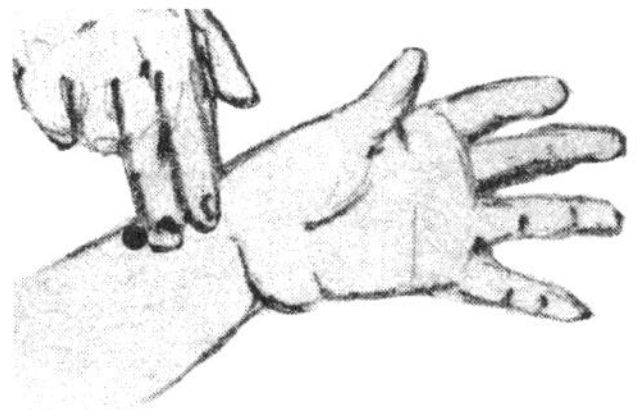

Figure 3

Chinese Massage[1]

1. Do this with the child lying face downward or sitting up with his back towards you. Place your fingers on the child's shoulders, over his clothing, and massage the fleshy areas above and between the shoulder blades. This has a strong relaxing effect, refreshes the entire system, and releases tension from the lungs (Figure B).

2. With your fingers, massage from the middle of the nose to the bottom of the ears, using gentle pressure. Cover the highest fleshy part of the cheeks. This clears the sinuses (Figure C).

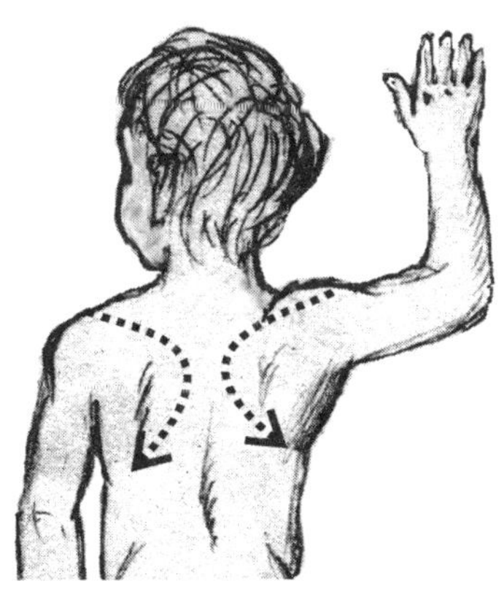

Figure B

Conclusion

Children with colds may easily switch from feeling warm to feeling cold and from being listless to being hyperactive. Generally speaking, a high fever passes quickly when children have a strong constitution. This indicates good health and a tendency to heal quickly. With care and suitable preventive measures, you can ensure your child's good health.

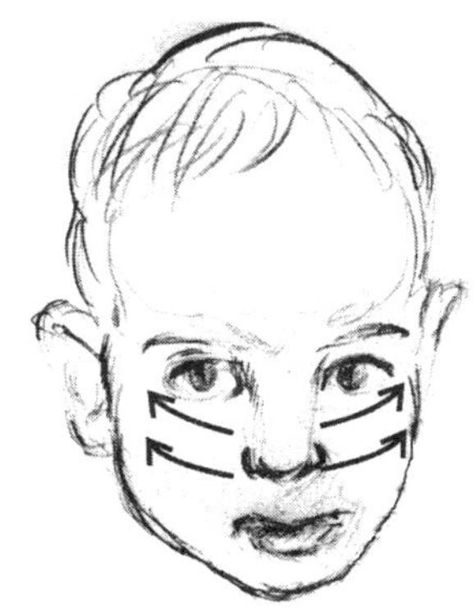

Figure C

137

---

[1] Russell and Gordon, pp. 36, 50.

Constipation in Children

In the section on constipation in adults (Chapter III), I mentioned that constipation causes many problems. This is valid for children too. However, the advice contained in this article is geared specifically toward children.

Causes

Nature and nurture

Constipation, especially the chronic type, is rarer among children than among adults. This is because adults are "more educated," or more to the point, badly educated. They are taught that they should not sit on lavatory seats in unknown places. Therefore, they refrain from using a bathroom when they need to, which makes the bowels lazy or dormant. This, in time, will lead to constipation. Since children are "less educated," they tend to be less constipated.

There are, though, some children who do suffer from constipation more than adults do. No doubt, these children have a physical propensity. However, one should not forget that tendencies have to be triggered to be active. It is therefore reasonable to assume that early training plays a part. The mother, who probably suffers from constipation herself, warns the child at an early age not to use the school toilet, but to wait until he gets home from school, fearing, perhaps justifiably, that the child will catch diarrhea or germs from other children. She may take her child on a trip lasting several days, during which both refrain from relieving themselves. So what is the stronger factor here – nature or nurture? This type of parent generally tends toward too early and too strict hygienic training. According to Freud, there are "anal-retentive" children, that is, their sexual and general energy (libido) is centered around the anus, and they consider feces their private property. They simply are afraid to let go of their feces or share them with others. Such children tend to grow into chronically constipated adults.

Poor toilet training

Constipation may occur in children as the result of poor toilet training. This process is difficult for both mother and child. The mother eagerly awaits the moment when the child will start using the potty. The child wants to
138

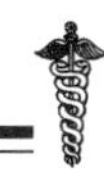

please the mother, but simply "cannot deliver the goods." This is when the serious problem begins. The child strains, which is painful, and then is afraid to try again, so he holds back. Sometimes, the child learns to control himself, but not to "let go." The mother then gets worked up, which makes the child more tense and thus a vicious cycle is set in motion resulting in chronic constipation.

Inadequate intake of fluids (babies)

This usually occurs during the summer months when nursing mothers might need to supplement their milk with other fluids. If the amount of liquid the baby consumes is insufficient, the result is dehydration and constipation.

Inadequate diet

The main cause of constipation is diet-related. Both the food itself and unhealthy eating habits play a part, as I shall explain.

Prevention

Constipation and its side effects, such as flatulence, hemorrhoids, nausea, and headaches, can be prevented by following these recommendations:

♦ ***Advice for nursing mothers:*** Nursing mothers who do not want to give their babies water or tea supplements should nurse their babies more frequently, and drink more to dilute their milk.

♦ ***Relaxation:*** Both mother and child should practice relaxation and openness.

♦ ***Appropriate toilet training:*** Toilet training at the right time and in a healthy and tolerant atmosphere will do much to prevent constipation.

♦ ***Regular toilet habits:*** The child should be trained to go to the bathroom each morning as soon as he gets up. According to Chinese medicine, the colon is ready to evacuate at this point.

♦ ***Correct eating habits:*** The child should have regular, leisurely meals and not indulge in hasty snacks. He should be taught to chew his food well and not overeat.

♦ ***Diet:*** Give your child plenty of vegetables, fruit, whole-grain cereal (such as whole-grain rice, whole-wheat bread), natural foods, and plenty of fluids. Supper should be light, served early, and include mainly vegetables (especially lettuce) and oats.

Treatments

Dietary remedies

♦ Soak dry fruit (especially prunes) overnight in water. The child should drink the juice on an empty stomach the following morning.

♦ In serious cases, and only once in a while, soak linseed overnight. This will form a jelly that may be added to yogurt. The child should eat the mixture on an empty stomach. (A salad dressed with olive oil and lemon and sprinkled with oats is also effective).

Watch for the foods that help relieve your child's constipation. Let the child eat wheat bran in yogurt and drink a lot.

Drinking plenty of fluids is very important. Allow the child to **drink** as much as he wants of the following: boiled water, water sweetened with honey, grapefruit juice, spinach juice, celery juice, and an equal mixture of beet and carrot juice.

Herbal remedies

The following mixture, which can be purchased in a health food store, is effective for relieving constipation:

Frangula (Buckthorn)

Salvia (Sage)

Plantago (Plantain)

Taraxacum (Dandelion)

Place a teaspoonful or two of the mixture in a cup. Pour boiling water over it and let it soak for 10 minutes. Strain and give it to the child to drink. A little honey may be added to sweeten the mixture. If this is too concentrated, add boiled water.

Massage

Massage olive oil into the child's stomach

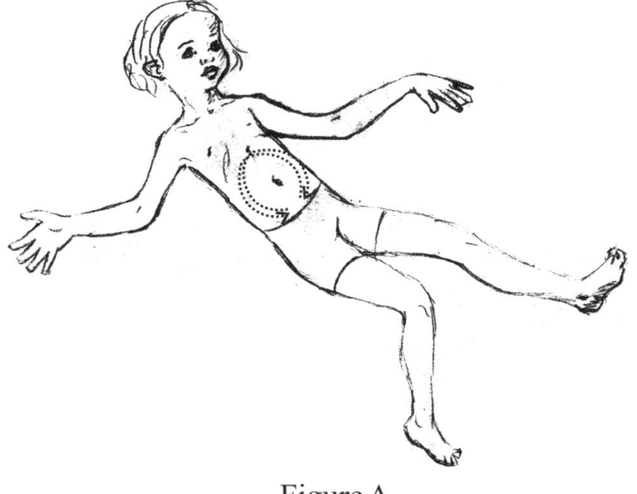

Figure A

140

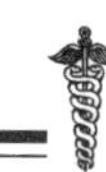

in a clockwise direction (the same direction as peristalsis). Stimulating peristalsis will help the child use the bathroom more frequently (Figure A).

Exercises

◆ Press the child's bent legs towards his stomach while he is lying on his back. Let go, and repeat. This activates the colon, and accelerates bowel movements. The child will cooperate more if you make a game of it.

◆ Play games such as "Ring around the Rosie" where the child goes round in a circle and suddenly sits down.

Natural laxatives (for babies)

If the above advice has not helped, take a parsley stem, remove the leaves, soak in olive oil or Vaseline, and insert in the child's rectum a number of times. This should not be done on a regular basis, since it may lead to "a lazy colon."

Reflexology

Give your child's feet a general massage. Press zones 23 and 21. Afterwards, press zones 36–28 on the right foot, and then 28–31 on the left foot (Figure B).

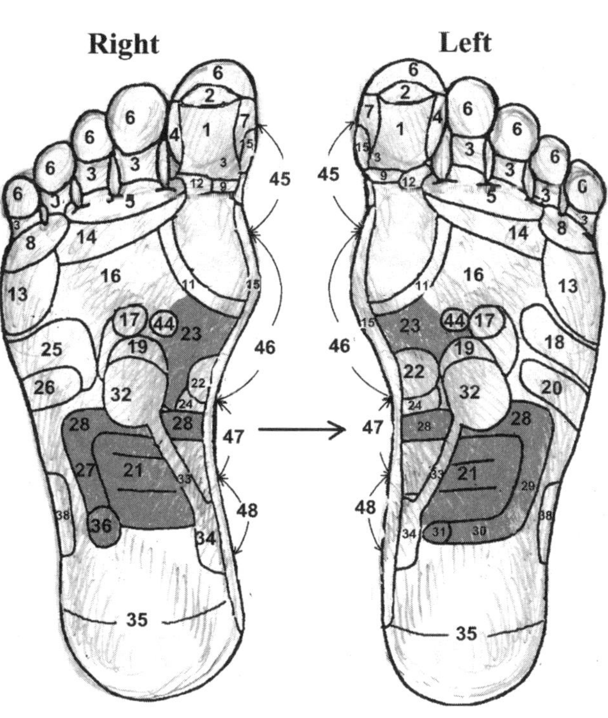

Figure B

Shiatsu

Shiatsu can help speed up sluggish or "lazy" peristalsis. The child should bend his legs, since this helps relax the constricted and painful tummy muscles, and breathe in and out rhythmically (synchronize your breathing with the child's). As you both breathe out, press down with four fingers starting with the clavicle and moving down the stomach to a point just below the navel.

141

Move along to the right side of the stomach, to the junction of the small intestine and colon (a little above the appendix). Move up along the ascending colon to a point to the right of the navel. Move across the navel along the transverse colon and down along the descending colon toward the left groin. An older child can learn to do it by himself (Figure C).

Note: The pressure should be applied while the child breathes out.

An older child can try shiatsu while on the toilet. The more pressure, the better the results. A footstool should be under the child's feet when he is sitting on the toilet.

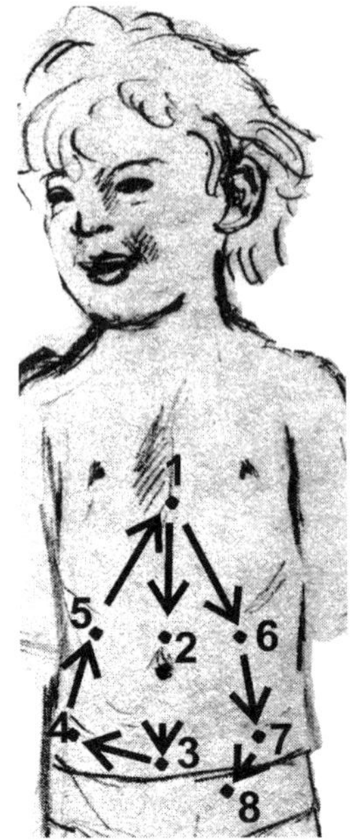

Figure C

Acupressure

Apply acupressure at each of the following four points. Fingerbreadth refers to the child's finger. Press down five times in succession, for about five seconds each time. Repeat this for a total of ten minutes.

1. The first point is situated in the soft tissue about four fingerbreadths below the lower edge of the kneecap, about one fingerbreadth away from the outer edge of the tibia (shinbone) (Figure 1).

2. The second point is on the outer part of the arm, about four fingerbreadths away from the wrist (Figure 2).

3. This point is situated just below the anklebone on the inside of the foot (Figure 3). You should keep pressing along the instep, until the edge of the big toe.

4. The last point lies on either side of the navel, about three fingerbreadths away from the navel (Figure 4).

There is no need to use all of the above remedies. Common sense should be applied to ascertain what helps your child most, in order both to cure him, and to prevent constipation in the future.

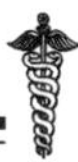

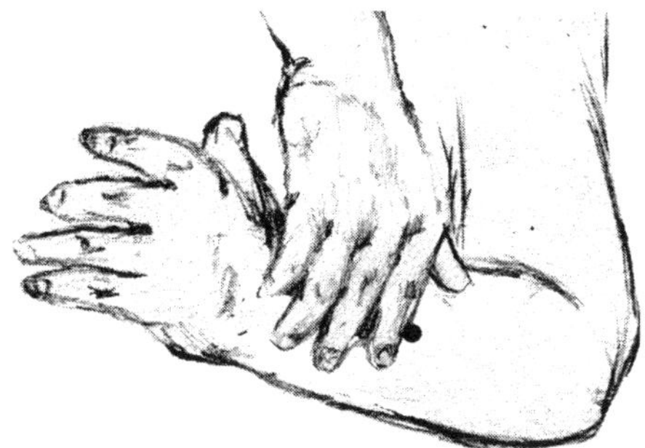

Figure 2

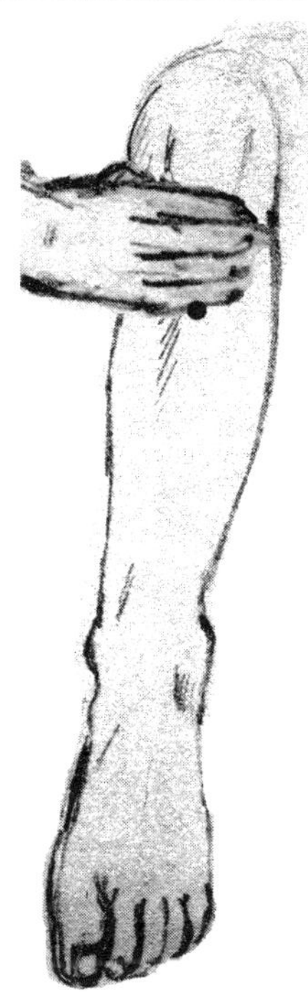

Figure 1

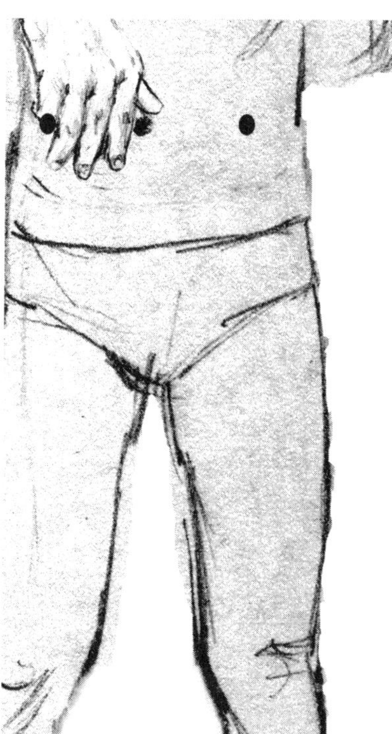

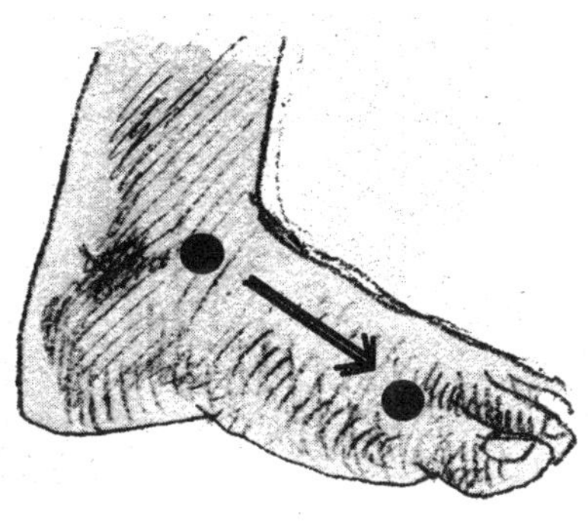

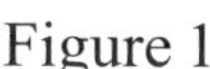

Figure 3

Figure 4

Diarrhea in Children

To this day I cannot forget a dispute that broke out between doctors in a hospital about whether to try and stop diarrhea in a baby who was losing weight daily. While two doctors favored using an infusion to stop the diarrhea — although they had not established the cause of it — a third doctor insisted on continuing to investigate the cause, claiming that the cause had to be found before starting treatment (he was certainly not sensible).

For the right approach, let's look to Chinese medicine. Chinese medicine, which uses common sense, says that sometimes the treatment itself points to the correct diagnosis depending on whether it works or not. We must not lose sight of the fact that our main concern is to heal, not to "be right."

While diarrhea is a health hazard for all, it is dangerous for the elderly, and can be fatal for babies and small children, due to the loss of fluid and the consequent risk of dehydration. Apart from fluids, the child may lose important minerals and salts, as well as "good" germs that help digest food. It is also harder to get a child to drink than an adult. Therefore, when diarrhea occurs in a generally healthy adult, we tend to allow the diarrhea to take its natural course and rid the body of the toxins that have accumulated, simply making sure that the patient drinks plenty of fluids. In the case of a baby, however, it is imperative to try and stop the diarrhea as soon as possible.

Much of the information in the section on diarrhea (in Chapter III) applies to children as well.

Causes

Diarrhea is a soft, watery bowel movement that is too frequent. Its color varies. Very cold food, fruit, fruit juices, colds, flu, germs passed on by other children, antibiotics, irritability, anxiety, etc. are possible causes of diarrhea.

A child may be sensitive or allergic to a certain antibiotic, to various foods such as milk, chocolate, ice-cream, cakes, certain types of vegetables such as cucumbers and tomatoes, or certain types of fruit such as watermelon or melon. All these may cause recurrent bouts of diarrhea in a child.

In addition, diarrhea may cause stomachaches accompanied by intestinal gas, stomach cramps, and discomfort around the anus. Even worse, it weakens the entire immune system, so that the child is prone to sinusitis,

144

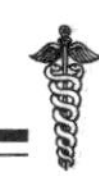

bronchitis, and asthma. This is borne out by Chinese medicine, which divides the energy lines and associated organs into pairs. In Chinese medicine the colon is paired with the lungs. Therefore, when the colon is playing up, watch out for the lungs and vice versa. Diarrhea may also be a symptom of illness, such as a cold or flu.

Prevention

In children, particularly in babies, diarrhea is very hard to prevent. Diarrhea may occur in babies as part of the digestive system's adjustment to life. However, once the child has recovered from an initial bout of diarrhea, the parents should try and trace the cause through a process of deduction. Try to discover whether anything unusual happened that day, or whether the child ate something different than usual. Remove the culprit from the child's diet and provide a substitute. For example, if cow's milk is the problem (as is often the case), use goat's milk or soya milk instead. Some food products have a laxative or allergic effect – that is, they create diarrhea, which is the body's attempt to "expel" them. I already mentioned some foods that fall into this category. For a complete list, a specialist in allergies should be consulted. Allergies are mysterious things: A simple food that very rarely causes problems may trigger a severe bout of diarrhea in one child. Sometimes a combination of foods, which if taken separately produce no negative reaction, can cause diarrhea. In such cases, it is extremely important to discover the cause. For more information, read the section on allergies (Chapter III).

Treatment

Diet

The first rule is to eat less and drink more. Initially, the child should be given rice water to drink. Take one cup of rice, wash it well, put it in a pan together with three cups of water, add a pinch of salt, boil for a short while, strain, and let the child drink it. After half a day or the following day, the child may eat the rice. The rice may be mixed with yogurt which contains acidophilus – an important digestive enzyme. Bananas, toast, boiled carrots, and a peeled apple are also effective. Children should be given plenty of blueberry juice, since it contains constrictive substances that help stop diarrhea. Coca-cola also contains constrictive substances, but consumption of it should be limited because of the gases it contains and because it may make the child hyperactive, when what he really needs is quiet and rest. Fluids and essential substances that are lost should be replenished by drinking boiled water with added salt and sugar, cocoa, and herbal teas (especially Mint, Sage, and Chamomile tea). Mint tea with lemon is useful for stomach or colon cramps, loss of appetite, hiccups, and halitosis.

The following remedies are helpful for older children with acute diarrhea. Soak an ordinary teabag in a quarter of a cup of boiling water for a few minutes. Open the teabag and empty its contents into the cup. The tea should be drunk together with the tea grains. It has a constrictive action that stops the diarrhea. If your child refuses to take this, try giving him a teaspoon of coffee and dry tea grains with a little sugar added. This mixture, recommended for older children only, "absorbs" fluids, and its constrictive action stops acute diarrhea.

Pomegranate juice is also effective and pomegranate peel even more so: Simply boil the peel for 10–20 minutes and give the child the water to drink after removing the peel. You can add a sweetener but not honey because it makes the diarrhea worse. If the child shows signs of dehydration (no tears, little saliva, or no urine) consult your family doctor or take him to an emergency clinic.

Once the diarrhea improves, the child may be given clear chicken soup to replenish the substances he has lost. Onion soup and oats also help strengthen the intestines.

Herbal remedies

A chronic loose bowel or chronic moderate diarrhea can be helped by this formula (after consulting a specialist):

Mix equal amounts of:

Quercus (Oak Bark) – excellent constrictive action

Chamomile – anti-flatulent

Fennel – anti-flatulent

Mint – constrictive action

Liquorice – good for the stomach

Place two teaspoons of the mixture in a cup, and add half a cup of boiling water. After letting the mixture soak for ten minutes, strain, and give the child to drink. (This method of preparation is known as infusion). If the tea is bitter, it can be sweetened, but not with honey.

This mixture can be prepared as a tincture. Give the child 30 drops in water, three times a day, on an empty stomach.

Reflexology

Massage first the left foot, from zone 31–28. Then massage from 28–36 on the right foot (Figure A).

Massage

Using olive oil, massage the stomach in a counter-clockwise direction. This halts the hyperactive peristalsis action (rhythmic movement of the wall of the alimentary canal) that causes diarrhea. While massaging, pinch the navel in a circular motion in a counter-clockwise direction (Figure B).

Acupressure

The following five acupressure points affect the digestive system and help stop diarrhea. Press gently or hard, depending on the child's response. Measure distances – fingerbreadths – using the child's fingers.

Press each point five times, for five seconds, and then repeat five times. This should be done five times a day. As the child's condition improves, reduce the number of "presses."

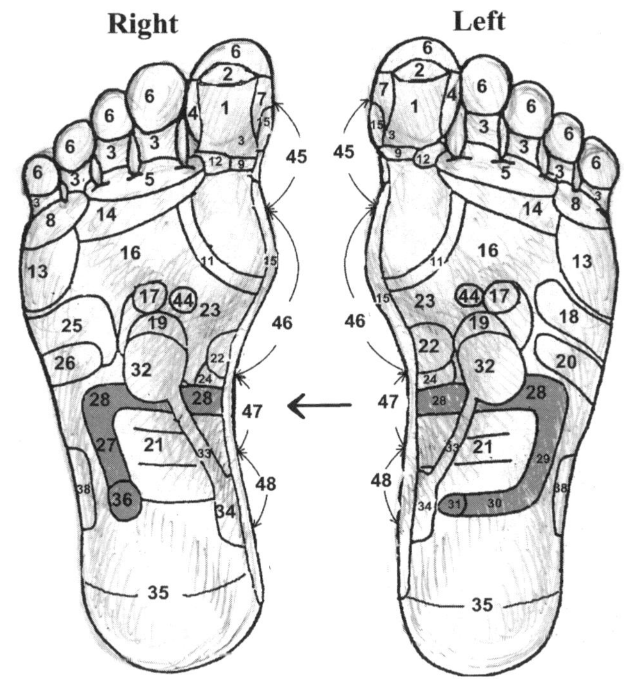

Figure A

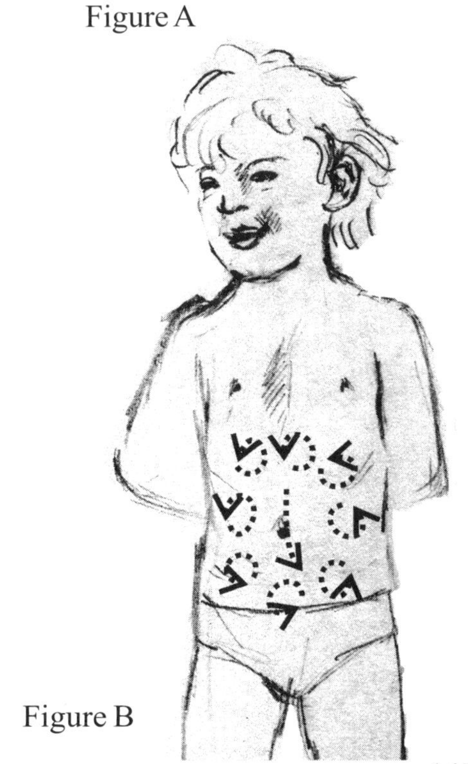

Figure B

1. The first point is known as colon 11: Find pressure point 1 on the elbow by bending your elbow and locating the external fold of the arm. The point lies at the edge of the fold (Figure 1).

2. This point is situated at the bottom of your toe on the inside of your foot. You should keep pressing along your instep, until you reach the bottom of your ankle (Figure 2).

3. The third point is on the hand between the first and second bones. Press down with your thumb hard toward the second bone of the hand (Figure 3).

4. The fourth point is located below the kneecap, 4 fingerbreadths down and 1 fingerbreadth outward. The child can be seated or lying down when pressure is applied. Use your thumb to press down, then massage in an upward direction (Figure 4).

5. This point is situated about 6 fingerbreadths above the navel, on the vertical axis of the stomach. With the child sitting or lying down, use your thumb or palm to massage, pressing inward (Figure 5).

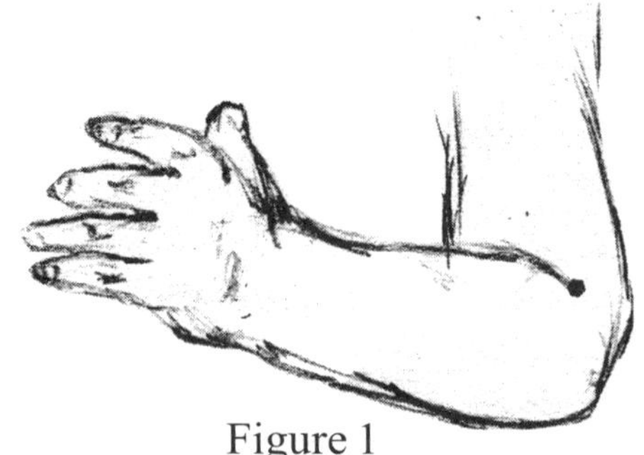

Figure 1

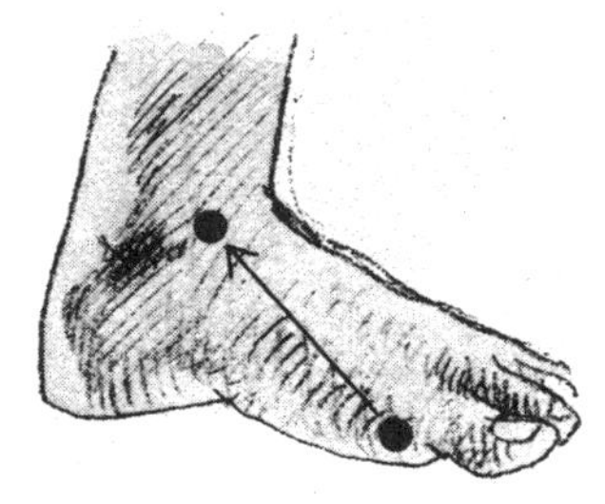

Figure 2

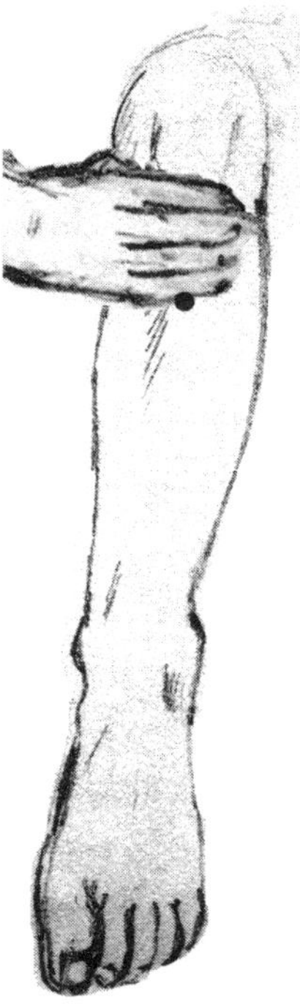
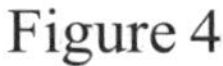

Figure 4

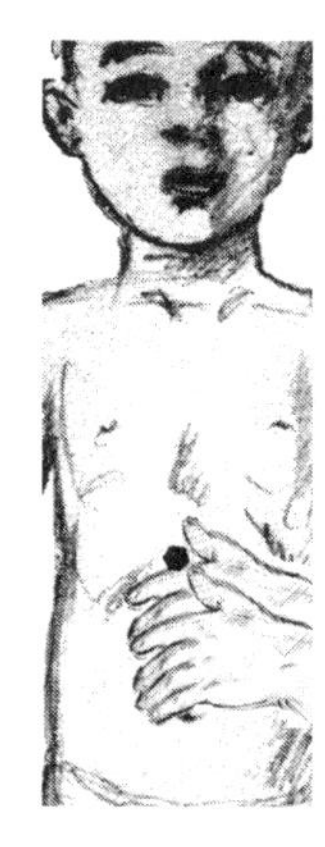

Figure 5

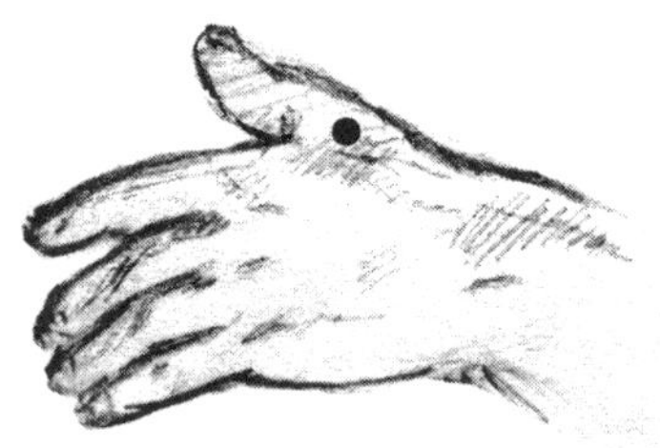

Figure 3

148

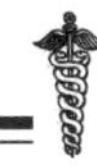

V. Nutrition:

Self-Healing Through Diet

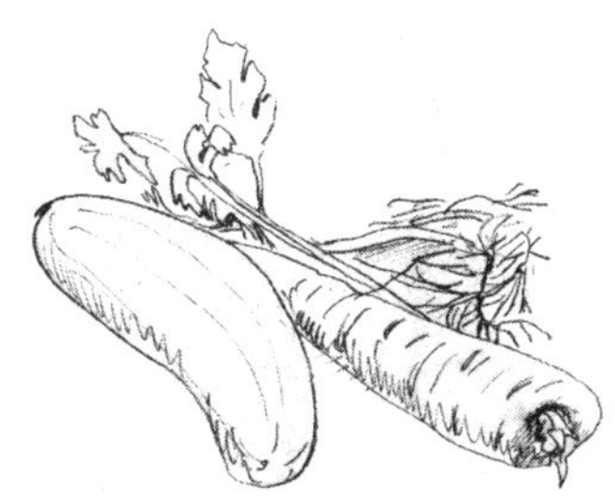

When discussing self-healing though diet, the key word is *self*, or you. Diet is simply one way of treating yourself. The illness is less important than what it indicates, and usually an illness indicates a personal history that has led to a state of imbalance or sickness. This history is linked to a combination of factors within you, which may include a genetically weak constitution (a weak immune system and low *jing* or essential energy) and "bad habits."

Sometimes poor eating habits learned in childhood may intensify a person's psychological problems, resulting in using food as a substitute for love or self- gratification, or in using food as a means of self destruction – eating foods you know are harmful, especially if you suffer from migraines or allergies. For example, crying babies are often nursed by their mothers or fed a bottle to calm them, not because the baby is hungry.

A Proper Diet

Even if you are healthy, it is important to consult an expert to determine what kind of diet is best for your particular needs. If you are not well, the same expert can help restore the body's natural balance through diet. "Ask your father and he will inform you, your elders and they will tell you." (Deuteronomy 32, 7) "Father" could mean a wise, mature person, and "elder" could mean an expert.

Be aware that drastic measures – such as fasting, enemas, or strict diets – without careful supervision can cause irreparable damage. Once, after several days on a diet, my daughter began to feel electrical impulses shooting through her body. She was momentarily unable to respond to what was going on around her and had difficulty in opening and closing her mouth. Fortunately, before any lasting damage was done, a doctor friend and I realized what was going on and stopped the diet.

As with all holistic medicine, the main goal is to treat the entire person – **you**, not just the illness or symptoms. To formulate the best treatment plan according to Eastern medicine, we need to determine your personality type; are you a *yin* or a *yang*, uninhibited or shy, nervous or easy-going? Is the illness, or the symptoms you are suffering from, the hot or cold type, in other words – acute or chronic? Is the problem one of surplus or deficiency, heat or cold, and so on. Cultural background and culturally influenced eating habits should also be taken into consideration.

This kind of assessment may result in some surprising discoveries. Let us say, for example, that you are an aggressive businessman, generally healthy even if a little on the heavy side, who travels a lot and often eats in restaurants. You will discover that your ulcer is very different from the ulcer your mother is suffering from. She is a frail, high-strung woman who is prone to insomnia and excessive perspiration. Obviously, to cure your ulcer, you will not adopt the same dietary changes that she will.

Three Approaches

To give you an idea of the breadth of concepts and suggestions that exist, I will briefly discuss three major approaches to diet and healing:
- The Jewish approach – based on the Rambam
- The Oriental approach – based on traditional Chinese medicine
- The Western approach

The Jewish Approach – the Rambam

The Jewish sources frequently mention the connection between food and healing. In the Talmud, *Tractate Berakhot* lists six foods that not only promote health, but that actually have healing properties – cabbage, spinach, honey, chamomile, tender veal, and liver. The Talmud differentiates between foods that prevent illness and foods that cure illness. Cabbage, for example, both prevents and cures illness, while spinach is more effective as a cure.

The Rambam, Rabbi Moshe Ben Maimon (Maimonedes), 1135–1204, was unique in both Jewish and medical studies. He was the royal physician in Egypt. The Rambam practiced and taught an individualized approach to medicine using extraordinary analysis and perception. The Rambam said

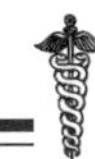

that his medical knowledge was based on two sources, Jewish tradition and Talmudic sources as passed down through the generations, and medical attitudes and principles that were common in his generation. These principles were usually passed down from father to son, or from physician to disciple, and were validated by medical geniuses of the time such as Gallinos and Hippocrates. He was aware of the connection between the soma and the psyche (the physical and the psychological). Gallinos healed the body, and the Rambam healed the soul.

The Rambam categorized foods according to their qualities, ranging from healthy to harmful. He recommended specific foods for hot-tempered people, for placid people, for children, and for the elderly. He described diets for various climates and seasons of the year, and the properties of various foods – hot versus cold foods, laxatives versus foods that constipate. The Rambam also discussed the order in which specific foods should be eaten; appetizer, main course, dessert.

When discussing foods that are most suitable for sick people, the Rambam emphasized the importance of finding a diet that *suits the specific ailment*. As for people who have a problem in a specific organ, or people who have been indulging in unhealthy habits for many years – "For each of these there are other ways and methods, depending on the sickness" (Rambam, *Hilkhot De'ot*, IV).

In an interesting essay on behavioral and psychological disorders, in Chapter Two of *Hilkhot De'ot*, the Rambam claims that disturbed people will often experience bitter as sweet and vice versa. Some may experience a craving for inedible substances such as earth or coal, and revulsion for tasty foods such as bread or meat, depending upon the illness. This is what Isaiah meant when he said, "They say of the bad that it is good, of the good that it is bad, they make the bitter sweet and the sweet bitter" (Isaiah 5:20).

According to the Rambam, when a person is not well, an extreme approach, such as fasting may be required as a temporary measure depending on the circumstances. He speaks not only of what we eat but also of how we live. A moderate way of life is not achieved through diet alone, but involves other aspects of lifestyle as well, such as physical exercise adapted to the individuals' needs and abilities.

In fact, the Rambam says that most illnesses are the result of eating too much, rather than not enough. He interprets the verse, "He who guards his mouth and tongue, guards his soul from troubles," (Proverbs 21:23) to mean that he who is careful not to eat the wrong foods, or speak badly of others, will be healthy in body and soul.

In general, the Rambam advocates the principle of moderation. He stresses the importance of a moderate diet and warns of the dangers of going to extremes, particularly if a person is healthy. He even advises against over-indulgence in "healthy" foods. "It is better to eat a little of harmful foods than a lot of healthy foods." For more detailed information on specific curative and preventative diets, refer to *Hilkhot De'ot*, Chapter Four, *Hanhagat ha'Beriut* (Regimen Sanitatis), and *Kitzur Shulhan Aruch*, Chapter 32.

It is not easy to apply the Rambam's dietary suggestions to our modern lives. Many of the foods he mentions are not the same as similarly named foods we are familiar with. For example, the radish he refers to is black with a very sharp flavor. The garlic he used is probably wild garlic, not the garden variety we use today. Foods have different names today and there are foods we have never heard of. According to one opinion, healing techniques discussed in the Talmud should not be applied in our times because people have changed.

Though it sounds as if we cannot use of much of the Rambam's wisdom due to historical and cultural differences, in fact, the *principles* remain the same. For example, what is essential is a diet suited to the needs of the individual, whatever his condition may be. We must also be careful not to automatically transplant diets from one type of climate and conditions to another climate and conditions.

The Oriental Approach – Traditional Chinese Medicine

According to traditional Chinese dietary theory, we get our basic or essential energy from two sources: the energy we inherit, and the energy that our body manufactures from what we eat, drink, and breathe. The food we eat fuels our daily activities and maintains our physical body. What we eat helps determine if we are calm, productive, fulfilled, and healthy, or if we, G-d forbid, burn out from stress and physical ailments.

The digestive tract is where the food we eat is processed and transformed into useable energy. The food must first be "cooked" to perfection in the stomach, which is like a cooking pot. The spleen is both the fire that heats the pot and the distillation mechanism that transforms the cooked food into useable energy. The stomach and spleen must both be in top operating form to provide nourishment that the body can assimilate and use effectively.

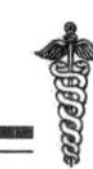

Cooking is like pre-digestion outside the body, making digestion in the body much easier. Less energy is required for the body to digest cooked food than raw food. Therefore, most people, most of the time, should eat cooked foods, since this makes the most efficient use of the energy available.

According to Chinese dietary theory, if the stomach and spleen are not able to perform their jobs adequately, sludge accumulates, just like what happens in a poorly functioning combustion engine. This sludge is stagnant food that has not been properly digested and is called dampness.

The concept of dampness explains a variety of functional difficulties that contribute to all sorts of pathologic problems. Dampness is the primary factor contributing to excess phlegm or mucous in the body. This inhibits the flow of life energy, as well as blood, throughout the body, and results in a variety of health problems for many people.

Besides eating mostly cooked foods, it is also important to know which foods have a dampening affect on your body – too much sweetness, especially in combination with sourness. In particular, excessive citrus fruit and juices, tomatoes, concentrated sweets such as sugar, molasses, and honey, and highly nutritional foods such as wheat, dairy products, nuts, oils, and fats create an overabundance of body fluids that become pathologic dampness. Cold or frozen foods and liquids also cause the stomach and spleen to work overtime and are not digested well. They should be avoided as much as possible. At the very least, do not drink cold liquids with your meals. Drink a small amount of warm water at mealtime, if necessary, and save the cold drinks for infrequent, between meal treats.

Certain combinations of food are worse than their individual parts. Put them together and you've got potential trouble. Ice cream is an example of a bad combination.

According to Chinese medicine, a cup of fruit juice is excessive nutrition and results in the formation of pathogenic dampness and phlegm. (It is interesting to note that until 50 years ago, nobody drank fruit juices. When left to sit, the juices fermented and were used for healing purposes.) Meat is also extremely rich in nutrition and therefore dampening. This doesn't mean you can never eat meat, only that you should eat it in minimal amounts.

In general, according to Chinese medicine, a healthy diet is made up of mostly complex carbohydrates and vegetables – with plenty of fiber. This means fewer animal proteins, refined sugars, oils, and fats. For most of us, this means a more traditional diet, a diet similar – at least in it's basic principles – to the well-known macrobiotic diet, or that of the Rambam.

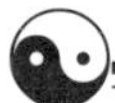

The Western Approach

If in Talmudic times, the issue of nutrition was complicated - despite medical traditions that were passed down through the generations - today, with constant new research, the issue has become infinitely more complex. Some of the numerous questions frequently asked include:

◆ Should I drink a lot or not?

◆ Is it better to eat one or two large meals or several smaller meals throughout the day?

◆ Should I eat a variety of foods at each meal, specific combinations of foods, or stick to only one kind of food per meal?

◆ Is it essential to eat all the basic nutrients at each meal or only some?

◆ Is garlic healthy or not? If yes, why did the Rambam discourage it?

◆ Are oranges and tomatoes healthy or not?

◆ What about the new studies that recommend drinking lots of orange juice when we were taught to drink only a little?

◆ Is milk healthy or not?

◆ Am I getting enough calcium?

◆ What about breakfast? We were all brought up to believe that a good breakfast was essential to a good day. So what's this new idea about eating only fruit until mid-day?

And above all,

◆ Which diet is the best?

If you are confused, you are not alone. With so much conflicting information, and new findings appearing on a daily basis, it seems ridiculous to deprive ourselves for twenty years only to be told that we could have eaten and enjoyed those foods in good health. After all, we live only once. As if all this were not enough, we are constantly being informed that almost every other product on the market is carcinogenic, according to reliable studies performed with control groups, using standard deviations, etc.

In view of all this, you may wonder if there is anything to eat that is not unhealthy. Don't worry, you won't die of hunger. On the contrary, you are more likely to die from overeating! The modern Western diet is a relatively recent result of post World War II advances in technology and transportation. Much of what is considered a normal diet is not healthy. Just as we have begun to realize that smoking, pollution, and high levels of stress are not healthy, we are also starting to realize that too much sugar, fat, oil, and animal proteins are also unhealthy.

There is not a shred of evidence to show that pesticides, preservatives,

154

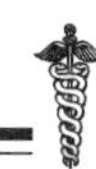

additives, and the assorted chemicals that are added to our food are health enhancing or health supporting. Our so-called convenience and fast foods are so filled with chemicals and have sat around for so long that there is often no nutritional value left in them. (I suspect that this is one of the reasons for the increasing frequency of cancer.)

The Western approach to diet varies from one type of diet to another, depending upon current research findings. However, there are some general principles that most practitioners agree with, especially regarding types of foods to avoid. These include caffeine, highly processed foods, heavy animal fats, salt, and dairy products. In general, everyone would benefit from a dampness-reducing diet as briefly described in the overview of diet according to Chinese medicine. This alone will help reduce many of the more common health problems that so many Westerners seem to suffer from. For specific problems and individual cases, it is best to consult a qualified practitioner.

Eat plenty of whole grains and fresh vegetables as well as moderate amounts of fruit, saltwater fish, lean poultry, and liquids. Below is a table of suggested foods you can easily and safely substitute for common foods that you may want to avoid.

Avoid	Why?	Acceptable Substitute
Caffeine	Stimulant	Herbal teas, hawayij,* grain coffee, ginger, cinnamon
Processed Foods	Harmful chemicals	Whole grain flours, breads, cereals, crackers, meals
White Sugar	Harmful chemicals	Molasses, maple syrup, honey
Dairy products	Create mucous	Soy or almond milk, almond butter, tofu
Salt	Causes fluid retention	Lemon or potassium salt

*Yemenite mixture of spices. Different mixtures are used for coffee and soup.

Remember – do everything in moderation.

Memory disturbances and amnesia among the elderly are not necessarily due to Alzheimer's disease or arteriosclerosis, but can also be caused by a vitamin B12 deficiency. Foods rich in vitamin B12 are mainly from animal sources – liver, fish, turkey, eggs, and dairy products. Vitamin B12 is also found in pickled vegetables, cabbage, beer hops, wheat germ, tempe (fermented soya), and miso.

I would like to emphasize two points. (1) The belief that only vegetarians and naturalists suffer from a deficiency in vitamin B12 is a myth. People who eat meat can also lack this vitamin; i.e. the deficiency is connected to the body's general nutrition. (2) It is worth noting that our bodies do not need large quantities of this vitamin. The small amount found in wheat germ and beer hops is sufficient. Mr. David Nachum, the president of the Israel Vegetarian and Vegan Society, tested this idea together with Mr. Mordechai Goren, a homeopath. For three months, he took a tablespoon of beer hops and a tablespoon of wheat germ, three times a day. During that period, the amount of B12 in his blood rose from 84 mg to 120 mg.

Man does not live on bread alone... (Deuteronomy 8:3)

I've written generally about different approaches to nutrition. Now I will provide more detailed information about some of the healthier food choices so that you can make informed decisions about how and what to eat or drink.

Liquids

After air, liquid is the most vital element for the physical survival of the body. People can live for a while without eating but not without drinking.

Liquids cleanse the body, help blood circulation, and have a calming effect. Drinking can also help and prevent diarrhea, constipation, migraines, dizziness, and many other symptoms. Consuming enough liquids is important for everyone, and especially for those suffering from low blood pressure.

How much should you drink is open to

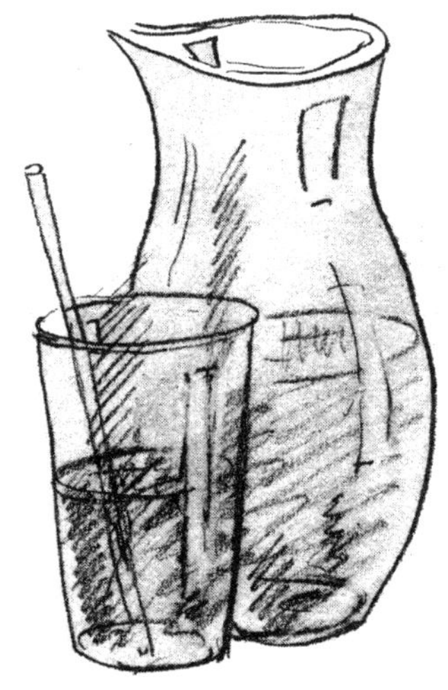

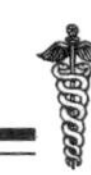

debate. Opinions vary and change. The Israeli Defense Forces used to enforce a strict water consumption regime. Today, however, the prevailing opinion is that liquid intake should be increased during physical exertion. The Chinese have a flexible attitude towards water consumption, taking into account the season and the temperament of the individual. An active person, more likely to perspire, should drink more, while a passive person who is less like to perspire needs to drink less. The Rambam had his own prescription, "Drink only when you are thirsty," but he was referring to a healthy person. The need to drink varies from person to person.

Each person must determine his or her own need for water. However, here are some general suggestions that apply to everyone.

♦ Do not drink during meals. The stomach needs acids for the digestive process and, by drinking, we dilute these acids and reduce their effectiveness. The Rambam advises against drinking water with food, but suggests that diluted wine might be useful especially for old people.

♦ Avoid all kinds of black coffee, tea, alcohol, and carbonated beverages or drinks that contain artificial additives or preservatives.

Drink mineral or boiled water, moderate amounts of natural fruit and vegetable juices, and above all, properly chosen herbal teas and infusions. In addition to being a pleasure to drink, herbal teas can be effective in treating a variety of problems.

♦ Passiflora or Linden tea is good for nervous people

♦ Peppermint tea is good for diarrhea

♦ Plantago tea is good for constipation

♦ Chamomile, Aniseed, Fennel, and Caraway seed are good for flatulence

♦ Crabapple or olive leaves are good for hypertension

♦ Rosemary tea will relieve symptoms of hypotension

♦ Hawayij for coffee can be added to all these infusions for its general tonic properties

Fruits and Vegetables

Many experts have stated that fruits and vegetables should be a basic part of a healthy diet, and I couldn't agree more. Fruits and vegetables are important for two reasons – their nutritional value and their purifying properties.

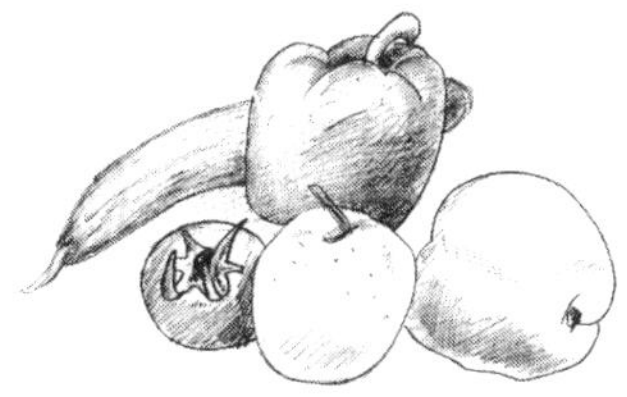

157

Fruits and vegetables provide vital nutritional substances that the body needs, as well as helping to collect and eliminate toxic wastes from the body. This prevents the accumulation of acidic waste which may turn into fat.

Fruit and vegetables are more effective cleansing agents than plain water because they combine their purification functions with a nutritional function. These two factors, paired together, in addition to obvious health benefits, can help make weight loss and maintenance easier.

All fruit should be cleansed thoroughly before eating to remove any chemicals that may have been used during the growing process. These chemicals can be dangerous to your health. Another note of caution: Fruit can be such an effective cleansing agent that it may cause diarrhea in some people. If this happens to you, remove the offending fruit from your diet for a while and then reintroduce it slowly. Some people even recommend fasting for a day. If fruit bothers you, you should be tested for sensitivity to fructose. The results of this test can help you plan a diet suited to your specific needs.

As an example of the old adage, "An apple a day keeps the doctor away," let me briefly list the health benefits that apples – only one example of fruit – provide. Apples are rich in vital minerals such as potassium, iron, sulfur, phosphorus, chlorine, magnesium, sodium, calcium, and also have a high Vitamin C content. Apples are effective in fighting against colds and against gingivitis (gum inflammation). They help fortify the body and calm the nerves. They are highly recommended as blood purifying agents. Apples are also good for the skin, liver, and kidneys.

Honey

Both Western and Eastern sources claim that honey is a highly nutritious and therapeutic substance. The Chinese grade honey according to its sweetness. Sweet honey, they claim, is nutritious and has both a tranquilizing and a tonic effect. According to the 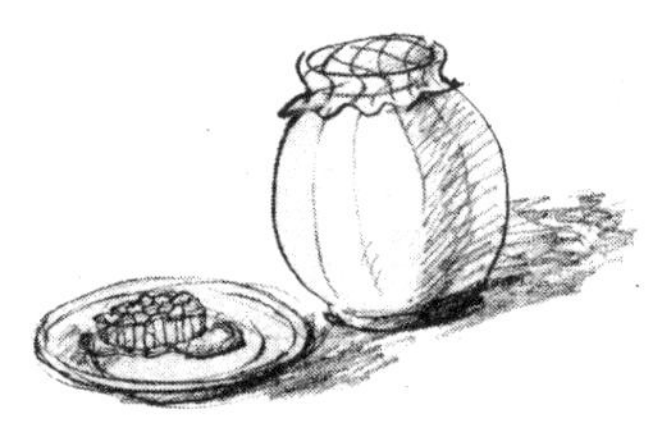 Rambam, honey is good for the elderly. In the West, honey is said to contain medicinal properties. It contains an active ingredient that is responsible for stimulating and activating vital life processes that help the body absorb sugar and derive maximum benefit from it. Others say that honey increases the supply of energy to the healthy heart and strengthens the weak heart.

Honey is beneficial to the digestive system by stimulating bowel movement and relaxing the stomach. (It is not recommended for a loose bowel.)

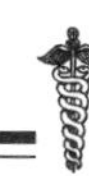

It also fortifies the liver, providing a source of fuel for this vital organ's functioning. It has prophylactic properties that help prevent colds and respiratory diseases. A mixture consisting of equal amounts of honey, onions, lemon, and brandy is a good cold remedy. (For children, use just honey and lemon.) (See section on Colds in Chapter III). Honey and horseradish syrup is a good cure for hoarseness. A mixture of honey and onions is an effective remedy for asthma. (See section on allergies in Chapter III).

Be careful – some people are allergic to honey.

Nuts, Seeds, and Dried Fruit

Vegetarians and advocates of natural foods eat nuts or seeds with almost every meal. They eat dried fruit frequently. This is not surprising, in view of the rich nutritional content of these foods. Not only do they taste good; they are important sources of the main nutrients; proteins, carbohydrates, fats, vitamins, and minerals.

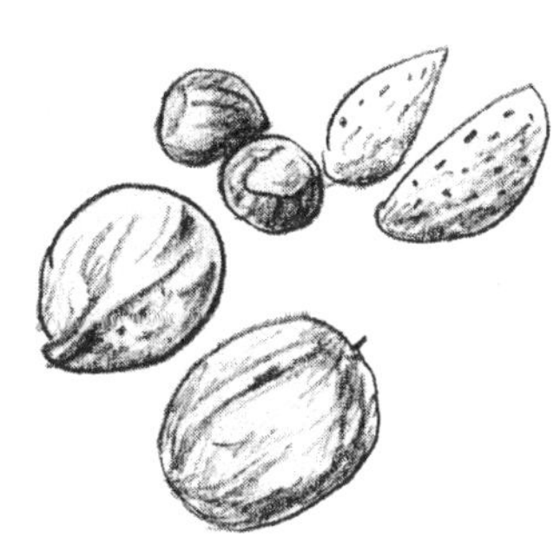

Walnuts, peanuts, almonds, and seeds contain polyunsaturated fats, which are both beneficial and therapeutic. Watermelon, pumpkin, and sunflower seeds are all rich in niacin, an essential vitamin in the B complex of vitamins. Almonds, walnuts, and peanuts all contain relatively high levels of protein, and almonds and walnuts – and especially unroasted pumpkin seeds – are thought to enhance sexual potency. Blanched almonds also relieve heartburn and absorb the acids and toxins connected to smoking. Nuts and seeds are also rich in calcium and iron – especially important for growing children. Young children should eat crushed nuts and seeds because of the danger of choking.

Almond milk (prepared by adding water to crushed almonds), nut and seed butters, and nut and dried fruit confections are highly nutritional. Almond milk can be consumed as a beverage or used in cooking and baking. Combine crushed almonds with date paste to make a simple and tasty confection. This can be rolled into balls and dusted with sesame seeds or ground coconut.

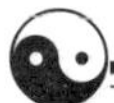

Garlic and Onions

Garlic is a universal food crossing all ethnic and class barriers. It can be found in gourmet cuisine and upscale restaurants. It is also found in the homemade recipes of our grandmothers who were aware of its beneficial properties long ago. Garlic is available in a variety of forms - fresh, crushed, powdered, paste, and even in tablets. Although tablets have the advantage of no odor, they leave out the unique,

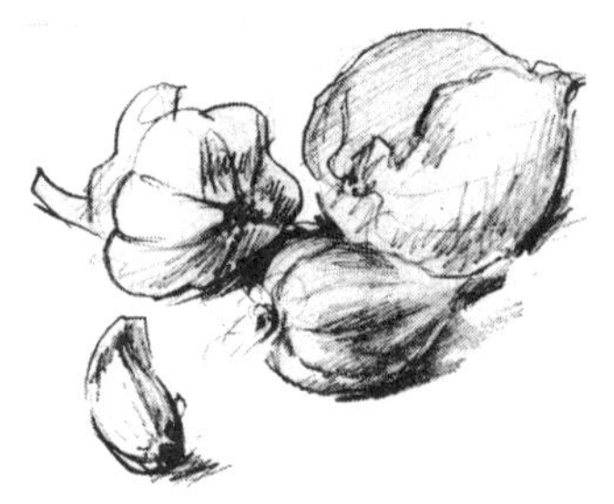

special flavor that has always been an integral part of good, traditionally prepared food.

In China the use of garlic is widespread. They recognize the fact – now also acknowledged in the West – that garlic purifies the blood, blood vessels, and intestines. It eliminates various parasites and helps urination. It facilitates proper breathing by preventing the accumulation of fluids and phlegm. It is also said to strengthen sperm.

The Rambam advised limited consumption of garlic, eating "small amounts during the rainy season only." One sage considered it an offensive food and demanded that those reeking of garlic leave the study hall. On the other hand, Ezra the scribe introduced a rabbinical regulation (*takanah*) that garlic should be eaten on Sabbath Eve since, "It fosters love, while quelling lust." During various time periods, the Jews were known as "garlic eaters" because they consumed more garlic than their gentile neighbors did.

The logical way to use garlic is in moderation. Eat it in moderate amounts together with other foods so that the body receives all the nutrients it needs. How can you eat garlic without becoming a social nuisance? The answer is simple. Eat fresh garlic with parsley or mint, and it will leave no odor.

Onions are similar to garlic in that all the properties of garlic also exist in onions, only in milder form. This mildness makes onions a good solution for breathing problems, asthma, etc. Since there is a link between asthma and allergies, onions are also effective in alleviating the symptoms of one of the problems that defies Western medicine – allergies.

Garlic and onions are healthy foods that should be eaten in moderation after steaming, cooking, or frying. Not only do they enhance the flavor of what you eat, but they also improve your health. That's a hard combination to beat.

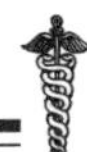

VI. A List of Medicinal Herbs and Their Use

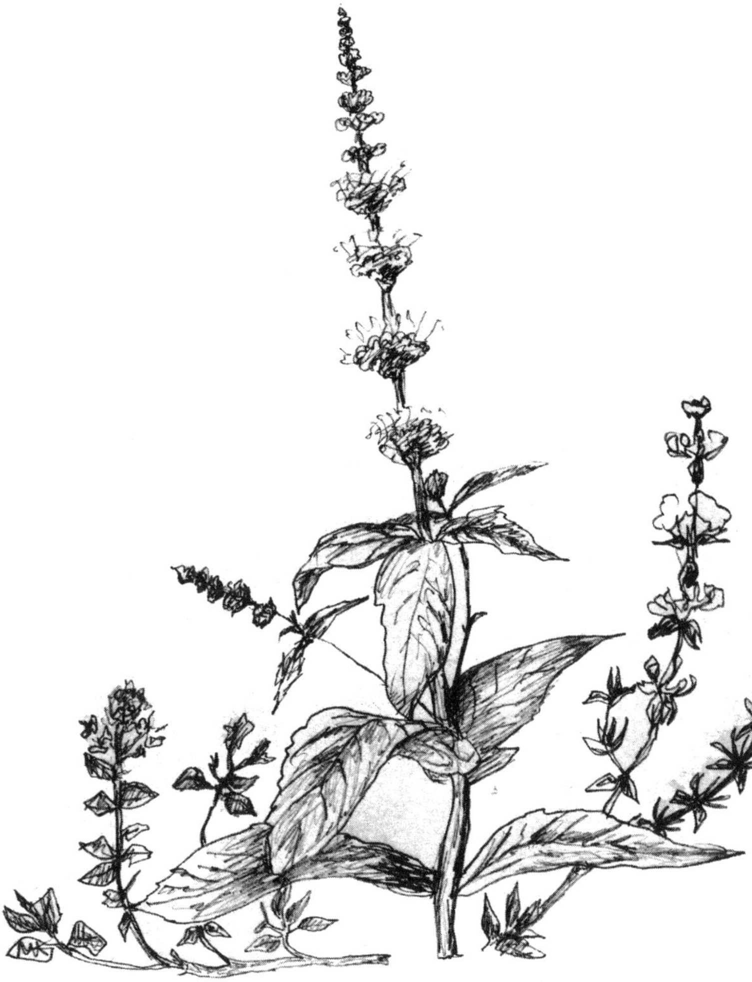

The lists below explain what each plant is used for. The herbs can be taken as tinctures (suspended in alcohol extract), syrup, infusion, or capsules. All should be taken on an empty stomach.

Note: People who suffer from heart problems, high blood pressure, diabetes, and other serious diseases should not use tinctures which are alcohol-based. Diabetics must also avoid syrups, which are usually mixed with sugar. For them, tea (infusion) is preferable. In all cases, it is recommended to consult with a specialist before taking medicinal herbs.

Dosages:
Tinctures: 30 drops in a shot glass of water, three times daily
Syrup: One teaspoon, three times daily
Infusion: One teaspoon of the dried plant in a cup, cover with boiling water, let stand for 10 minutes, strain, and drink the liquid, three times daily.

Western Herbs
Because the Chinese herbs are difficult to find and to prepare, I will list only the Western herbs.

Respiratory System
For shortage of breath, coughs, or colds, take:

Echinacea (Cone Flower)	anti-inflammatory, against colds
Equisetum (Horsetail)	anti-allergic
Eucalyptus	antiseptic (against bacteria and viruses)
Louisa (Lemon Lipia)	effective against chills
Salvia (Sage)	effective against chills
Hydrastis (Golden Seal)	anti-inflammatory, dries mucous (should be avoided during pregnancy)

Musculo-Skeletal System
When back, neck, and/or joint pains disturb sleep, take:

Hamamelis (Witch Hazel)	compress for veins and muscular cramping
Harpagophytum (Devils Claw)	anti-diuretic
Hypericum (St John Wort)	nervous pains, coughs
Arnica	muscle pain (for external use, not near open wounds.)
Ruta (Rue)	muscle pain

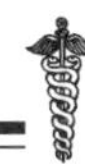

Digestive System

When digestive problems disturb sleep, the following have a pacifying effect:

Aloe Vera (Aloe)	constipation
Mentha (Peppermint	diarrhea
Senna (Cassia)	constipation
Frangula (Buckthorn	constipation
Foeniculum (Fennel)	flatulence
Filipendula (Meadowsweet)	reduces stomach acidity
Anis (Aniseed)	flatulence
Lavendula (Lavender)	digestion, flatulence
Chamomilla (Chamomile)	flatulence
Cardamonum (Cardamon)	flatulence

Skin

For itching and related external problems (for external use):

Calendula (Marigold)	itching, burns, wounds
Plantago (Plantain)	hemorrhoids, cuts
Aloe Vera (Aloe)	burns, sunburn, insect bites

Blood

The following cleanse the blood, ridding the body of toxins. For a purifying effect:

Calendula (Marigold)	anti-inflammatory
Viola - Tricolor (Pansy)	eczema
Taraxacum (Dandelion)	anti-inflammatory
Arctium Lappa (Burdock)	psoriasis
Urtica (Nettle)	eczema

Vascular System

For heart and blood pressure problems, use:

Crataegus (Hawthorn Berries)	blood pressure (mainly), irritability, strengthens heart
Vescum alba (Mistletoe)	blood pressure (secondary), irritability
Digitalis (Foxglove)	strengthens heart, blood insufficiency

Urinary System

Instead of running to the bathroom all night, take the following herbs to strengthen the urinary system.

Uva Ursi (Blueberry)
Betula Alba (Silver Birch)
Urtica (Nettle)   also helpful for skin problems
Agasthoma (Buchu)   antiseptic
Salyx Alba (White Willow)
Arctium Lappa (Burdock)

Immune System

When recurrent illnesses disturb sleep, the following are helpful to strengthen the immune system.

Echinacea (Cone Flower)
Alfalfa (Lucerne)
Propolis
Achilea (Yarrow)
Taraxacum (Dandelion)
Pollen

Reproductive System

In addition to the herbs for the immune system, use herbs from the following list:

Eleutherococcus (Siberian Ginseng)   strengthening
Turnera (Damiana)   strengthening
Gota-Cola   stimulating
Urtica seeds (Nettle)   stimulant, tonic

Herbs with tranquilizing effects

Passiflora (Passion Flower)   excellent tranquilizer with no side
                                                              effects
Melissa (Balm)   tranquilizing effect
Scutellaria (Skullcap)   tranquilizing effect
Humulus Lupulus (Hops)   tranquilizing effect
Valeriana (Valerian)   induces sleep

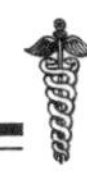

VII. Orthopedic Exercises for the Neck, Hands, Shoulders, Upper and Lower Back, Ankles, and Knees

*Compiled by Aryeh Krashinski, M.A.,
qualified in acupressure and Chinese massage.*

Preliminary Basic Guidelines for Orthopedic Exercises

Rising from a sitting position: Place your hands on your thighs.

Rising from a lying position (on a bed, etc.)**:** Lie on your side, lower your legs to the floor and push your body up, using your hand.

Getting up from the floor: First kneel, raise one leg to an angle of 90 degrees, and then stand up. If you find this hard, you may use a chair to help lift yourself up.

Pain: Do not do the exercises if you are suffering from serious pain.

If you suffer from a backache, avoid strenuous or rapid exercise (including an exercise bicycle).

Lying down: Try and sleep on a hard (preferably orthopedic) mattress.

1. You should sleep on your side (the natural position for sleeping) with a cushion between your knees and under your head.

2. When lying on your back, place a rolled up towel under your neck (preferably an orthopedic cushion which can be purchased at a pharmacy). Do not forget to place a cushion under your knees.

3. If you experience backache when lying on your stomach, try placing a cushion below your pelvis (reduces pressure on your spine). You can also place a cushion under your ankles.

4. You may lie with one knee pulled up – in a fetal position.

Lifting objects: When lifting an object, stand near the object, keeping your back straight, bend your knees (you should be using your leg muscles, not your back muscles) and lift with the object held close to your body.

Correct sitting or standing posture: Keep your back straight. Correct posture maintains the natural hollow in the lower back. Incorrect posture leads to lordosis (curvature of the spine) and places pressure on the spine, which causes backaches.

1. Preferably sit on a chair with a solid back, and sit straight against the back of the chair. Place a cushion or rolled up towel against the hollow of your lower back.

2. When sitting down or getting up from a chair, keep your back straight, do not lean forward.

3. When sitting in a car, keep your back straight and against the back of the seat.

Sitting at a desk: Make sure you have a suitable chair and that it is positioned near the desk. Sit up straight. If the chair is high, use a footrest to ensure that your thighs are at the correct height.

Flatfeet: Flatfeet can cause backache. Go to an orthopedist to be fitted for insoles.

Air-conditioning: Cold air arrests energy flow in the body and causes rheumatic and joint pains, as well as muscle cramps. People with backaches should avoid air-conditioned rooms.

General notes:

♦ Begin each exercise with a deep intake of breath and exhale during the exercise, unless otherwise specified.

♦ If you suffer from severe pain that makes it hard for you to walk or stand up, you should not be doing the exercises, but should be resting instead..

♦ Each exercise should be performed up to the pain threshold.

♦ If an exercise causes you severe pain, skip it.

♦ Any exercises you skipped due to pain can be performed the following day.

♦ Repeat each exercise 5–10 times unless otherwise stated (always inhale and exhale as described above).

♦ The exercises need not be performed daily. You can reserve certain

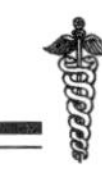

exercises for specific days (e.g. neck exercises for Sundays, etc.).

◆ Always rest between exercises.

◆ Do not stand immobile for any length of time, do relaxation exercises.

A. Warming-up exercises (standing)

These exercises are suitable for all types of problems. You may do as many or as few as you wish.

1. Lift your arms to an angle of 90 degrees and move your hands up and down (a form of greeting).

2. Raise your forearms towards your shoulders and drop them.

3. Raise your shoulders toward your ears ("shrugging" gesture).

4. Throw your right arm over toward your left hip while exhaling. Do this five times. Repeat with the other arm in the opposite direction.

5. Rub your arms to open the meridians and get the energy flowing.

6. Get the energy flowing in your fingers. Starting with your little finger, bend it forwards and backwards. Press along the length of the little finger on both sides, and front and back. Complete the exercise by pulling your little finger. Repeat with each finger. The thumb should be bent forward, backward, and sideways, too. Switch hands. (According to Chinese medicine, this eliminates bad energy through the fingers).

7. Tap lightly on your skull with your fingers to get the energy flowing in your head (this acts as a general tonic, as well as improving memory).

Begin by tapping along the central axis of the skull, from the forehead to the back of the neck. Repeat on either side. End with light taps on the forehead toward the temples and the back of the neck.

8. Shake your arms and hand to release and eliminate bad energy.

B. Neck, arms, hands, shoulders, and upper back exercises

Hand and wrist exercises (for those suffering from rheumatism)

1. Add a handful of sodium bicarbonate, coarse salt, or Epsom salts to a bowl of lukewarm water. Soak your hands and move them around in the solution.

Fingers: Bend your fingers as far as they will go and straighten them completely.

2. Thumb: Bend your thumb over toward the base of your little finger

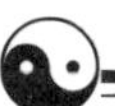

and then in the opposite direction until your fingers are splayed.

Neck exercises (standing up)

Note: Between each exercise, free the neck and head by shaking your head loosely to the right and to the left.

3. Stand straight and, with your face and eyes facing forward, stretch your neck up as far as it will go. Do not lift your chin. Stretch your head forward and your shoulders back. Return to original position.

4. Standing straight, stretch your neck up, and bend your head alternately to the right and left. Stretch your head and shoulders first to the right and then to the left.

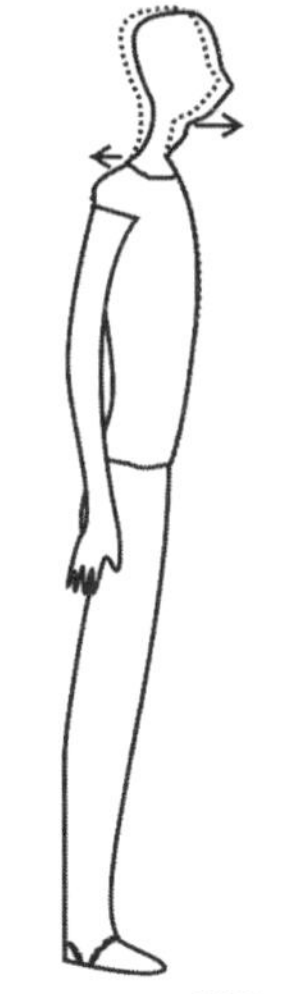

B3.

5. Stand straight and stretch your neck up as far as it will go. Place your balled fists under your chin and push your head as far back as it will go against resistance of the neck muscles.

6. Place your elbows and lower arms against each other with your elbows close to your body. Lift your arms up as far as possible, breathing in deeply. Return to original position, exhaling.

7. Stand with your neck stretched upwards as far as possible. Turn your head to the left and press your chin into your left shoulder. Move your chin toward the right shoulder by moving it across your chest. Move your chin back to the left shoulder (top of the shoulder) and repeat three times. Repeat three times in the opposite direction.

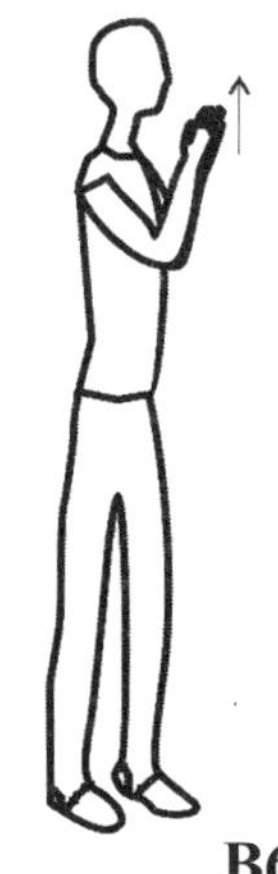

B6.

8. Stand with your neck stretched up and chin tucked in. Turn your head alternately to the right and left . When turning your head to the right, use your right hand to massage and press on the muscles of the left shoulder, and vice versa when you turn your head to the left.

9. Ear to shoulder – bend your head toward your shoulder and back. Repeat on the other side. Do this exercise three times.

Shoulder and upper back exercises (standing)

Note: If you feel tired between these exercises, per-

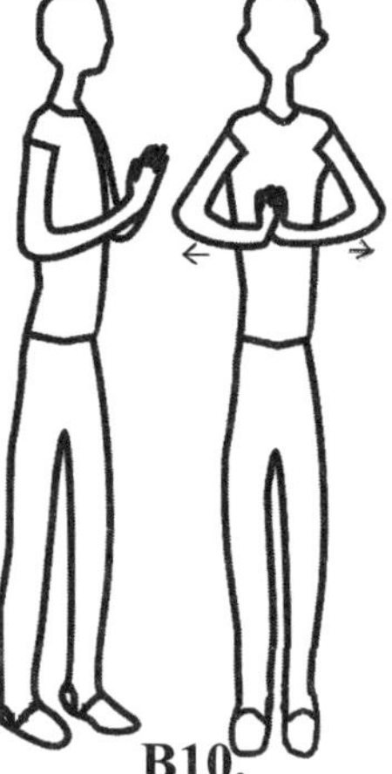

B10.

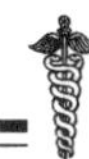

form the neck exercises described above.

10. Stand with your feet slightly apart, hands joined, fingers straight and pointing upward. Move your arms and elbows alternately to the left and right as far as they will go. Resist the movement with the other hand.

11. Stand with your feet slightly apart and hands hanging down at your sides.

a. Rotate your shoulders backward, (raise them up, back, down, and forward) 5–10 times.

b. Rotate your shoulders forward (up, forward, down, and back) 5–10 times.

c. Rotate your shoulders back (see a. above) 5–10 times.

12. Stand with your feet slightly apart and arms hanging down. Lift your right hand forward and upwards, stretching your fingers as far as they will go. As you lift your hand, rise onto your toes too. Repeat with your left hand breathing in when lifting your hand, and breathing out when lowering it.

13. Stand with your feet slightly apart. Link your fingers with the palms facing outwards, and stretch your arms forward and upward. Follow the movement of your arms with your eyes. As you raise your arms, rise onto your toes, inhale deeply when lifting your arms, and exhale when lowering them.

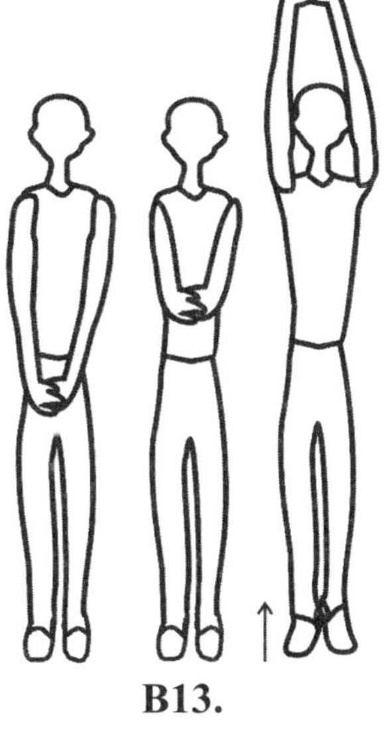

B13.

14. Stand with your feet slightly apart and arms loose by your sides. Lift your arms, palms facing down and lower them. Lift your arms above your head, palms facing inwards and follow the movement of

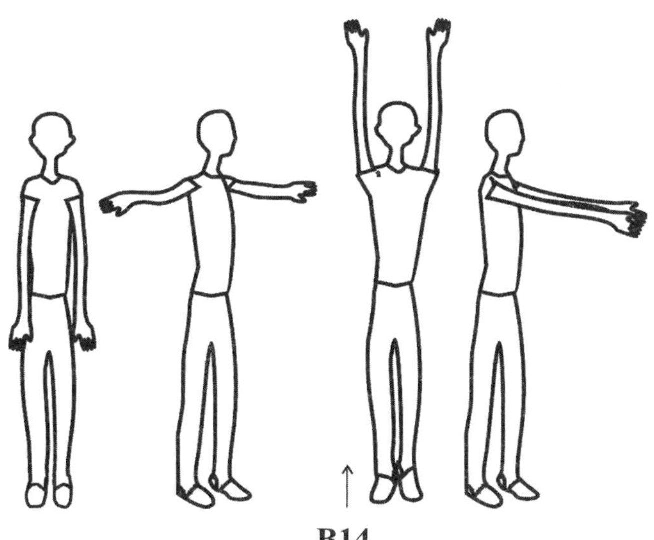

B14.

your arms with your eyes. Stand on to your toes and lower your arms to your sides, breathe in when lifting your arms, and out when lowering them.

Shoulder, neck, and back exercises using a meter-length rod

15. Stand with your feet slightly apart and your arms hanging down. Hold the ends of the rod and, with your arms straight, move it from right to left and vice versa.

16. Stand with your feet slightly apart. Hold the ends of the rod, lift your arms, and, holding them straight, move the rod from right to left and vice versa.

17. Stand with your feet slightly apart and arms straight by your sides. Take hold of the rod and, bending your arms, lift the rod to your chest, straight up, over your face and move it toward the back of your neck up to the threshold of pain. Return the rod to its original position.

18. Standing with your feet slightly apart, place the rod behind your bottom. Hold the rod at either end and, with your arms straight, move it from right to left.

19. Standing with your feet slightly apart, and your arms straight by your sides, place the rod behind your bottom. Keeping your back straight, bend your arms behind you up toward your back, and lower them. Keeping your arms straight, raise them behind your back to the threshold of pain and return to your original position.

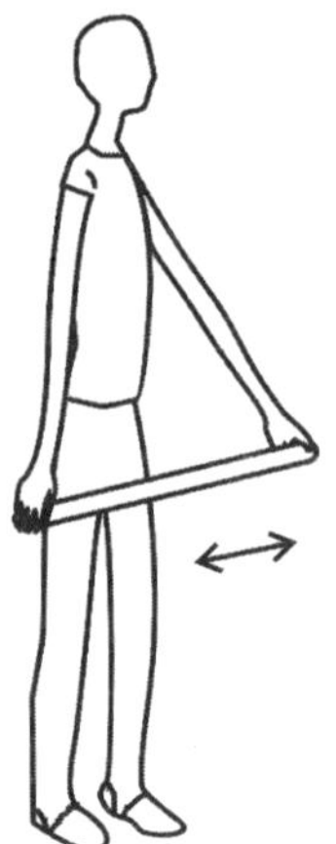

B15.

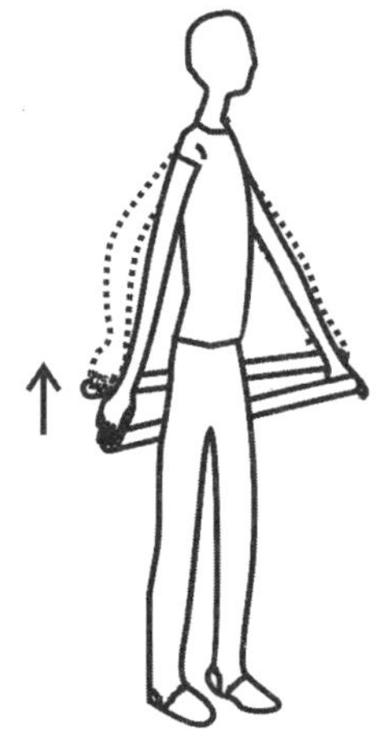

B19.

C. Lower back exercises

On your back

1. Lying on your back with your knees as far apart as possible and your hands along your sides, move your pelvis from side to side, while keeping the lower back as close to the mattress as possible.

2. Lying on your back with your arms along

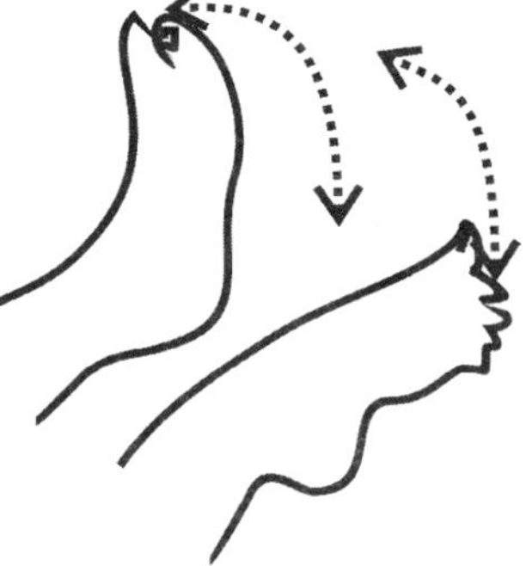

170

C2.

your sides, point your feet in opposite directions (down and up). Hold each position for five seconds.

3. Lying on your back with your knees bent, raise your bottom while contracting your stomach muscles. Leave your lower back against the mattress. Lower your bottom to the mattress, hold for five seconds.

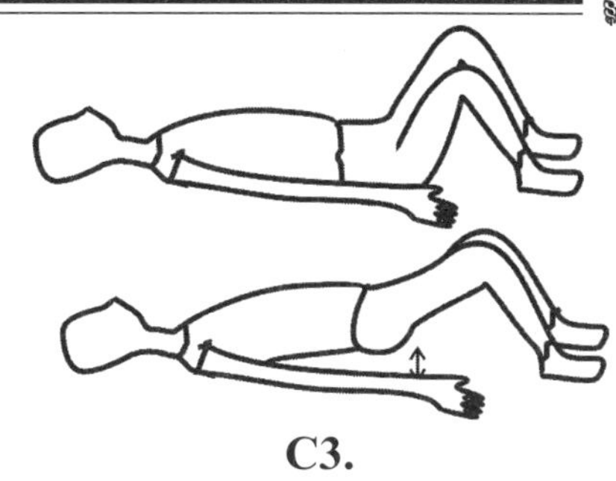

C3.

4. Lying on your back with your hands under your neck and knees bent, move your knees from side to side, inhale when your knees are in the center, and exhale as you move them to the side.

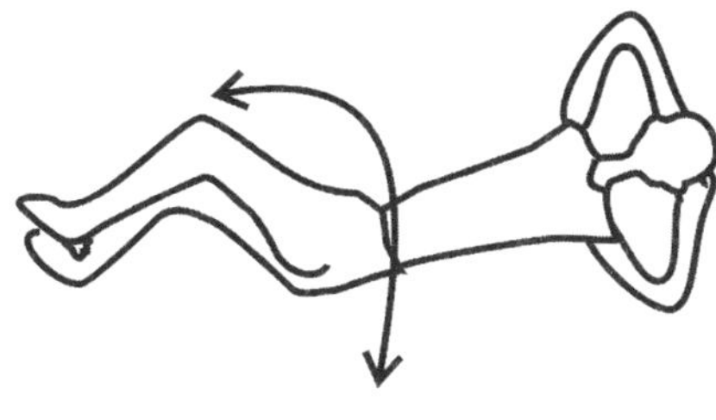

C4.

5. Lie on your back with your hands under your neck. Keep one leg straight and bend the other leg across the knee of the straight leg. Curve your body toward the bent leg. Switch sides.

6. Lying on your back with your hands under your neck and your knees bent, contract your stomach muscles and lift yourself up with your hands toward your knees while breathing in and out. Return to a lying position.

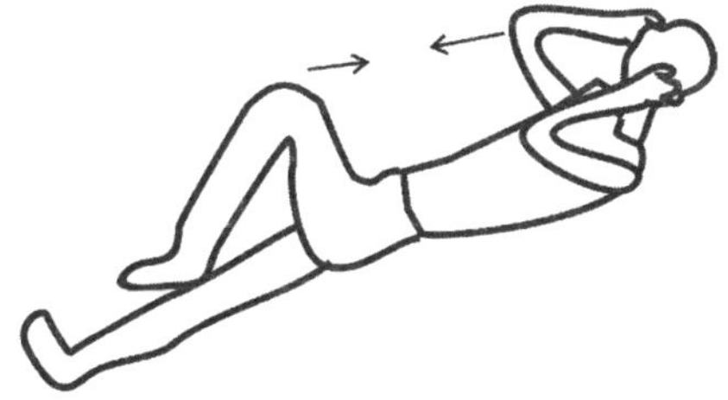

C5.

7. Lying on your back with your hands under your neck and knees bent, raise your right elbow toward your left knee and vice versa.

8. To prevent cramps after the two previous exercises (6 and 7), lie on your back with one leg straight and the other bent. Pull the bent knee in to your chest with 3–4 tugs. Switch sides.

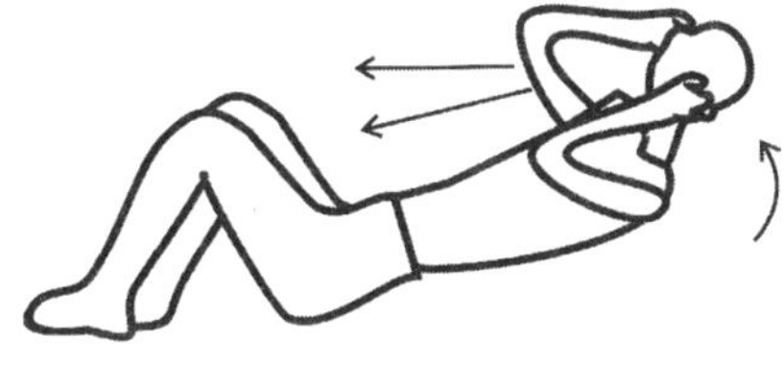

C7.

9. Lie on your back with your knees bent and pull your knees toward your chest, with 3–4 tugs of your hands.

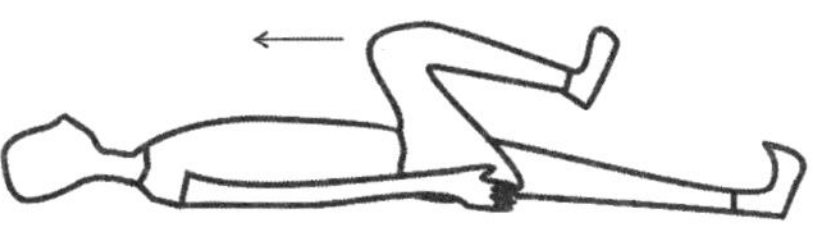

C8.

171

Return to original position.

On your stomach

10. Lie on your stomach with your toes pointing toward your head. With your arms bent and hands flat on either side, lift the upper part of your body about 5–30 times. For part of this exercise, turn your head to the right and then to the left.

11. To prevent cramps, do the last two back exercises (8 and 9) above.

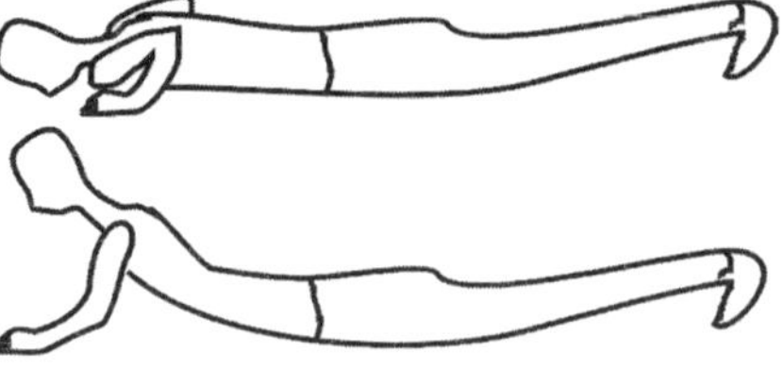

C10.

On all fours

12. Raise your head as far as possible and press down with your stomach as far as possible. Bend your head down and arch your back at the same time.

13. Position yourself on all fours. Sit back on your heels and stretch your arms and head forward. Return to original position.

14. Kneeling on all fours, move your right foot back until it is straight, hold for five seconds. Switch feet.

15. Kneeling on all fours, lift your right arm straight up toward your ear. Switch sides.

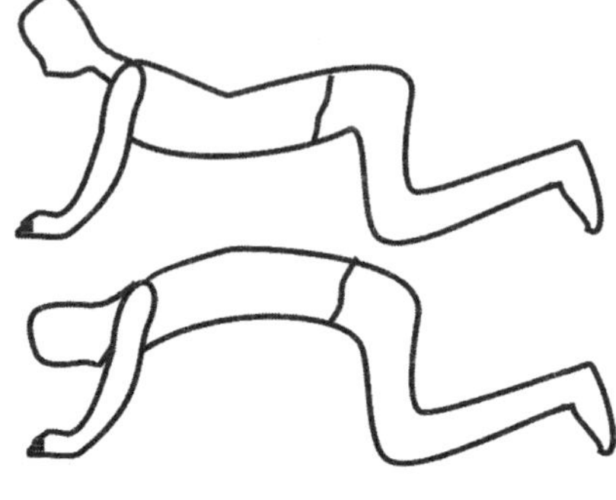

C12.

D. Ankle and knee exercises

On your back

Note: Between each exercise, shake your feet to both sides and up and down in order to relax the foot muscles.

1. Point your feet to either side in opposite directions, breathing out.

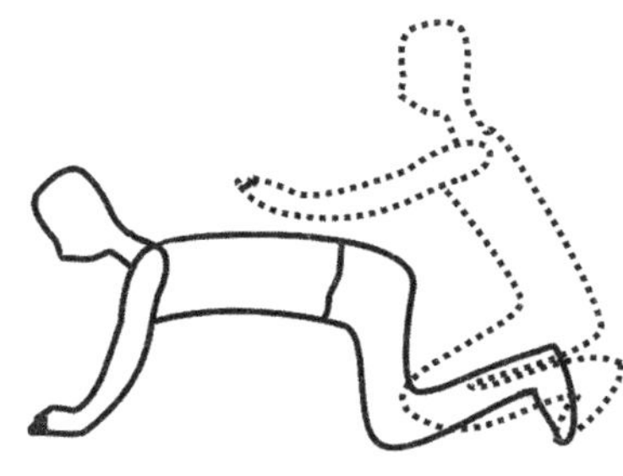

C13.

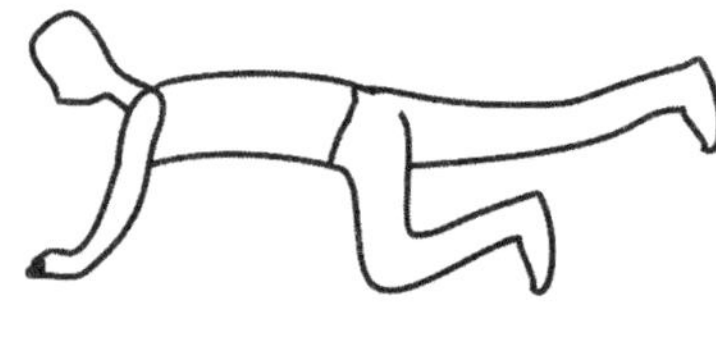

C14.

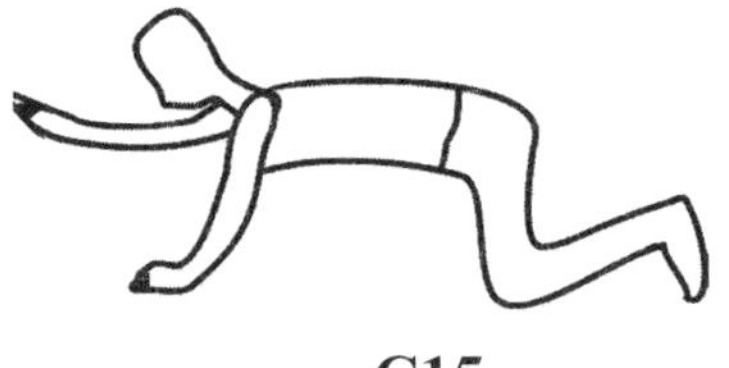

C15.

172

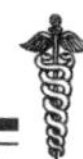

Hold for 3–5 seconds, and then change sides.

2. Point your feet toward you, hold for 3–5 seconds, and out, hold for 3–5 seconds.

3. Rotate your feet inwards.

4. Rotate your feet outwards.

5. With one knee bent, the other straight, with your toes pointing towards your head, press the straight knee down on the mattress (your heel will rise slightly). Hold for 3–5 seconds. Change sides.

6. With one knee bent, the other straight, and the toes pointing towards your head, stretch the straight leg, lift it up to a height of about 20 centimeters, hold for 3–5 seconds, and slowly lower. Switch sides.

7. With both knees bent, draw your knees up (pull them with your hands) toward your chest and back.

8. With one leg bent up and the other straight, perform a cycling motion.

On your stomach

9. Leaning on your toes, raise your knees and bottom off the mattress, keeping both legs straight, hold for five seconds.

10. Raise left leg to a height of about 20 centimeters. Switch legs (strengthens buttock muscles).

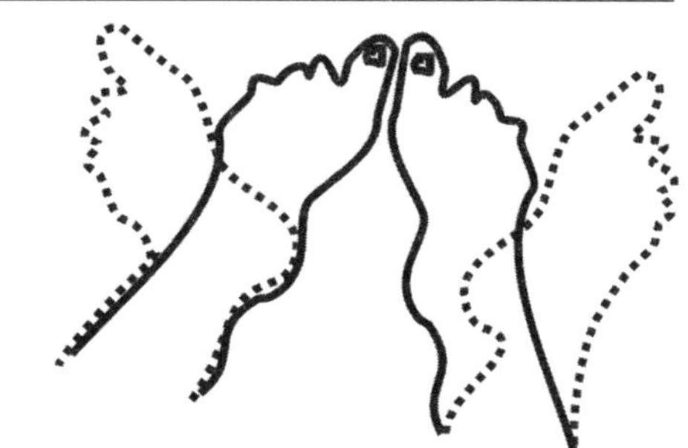

D1.

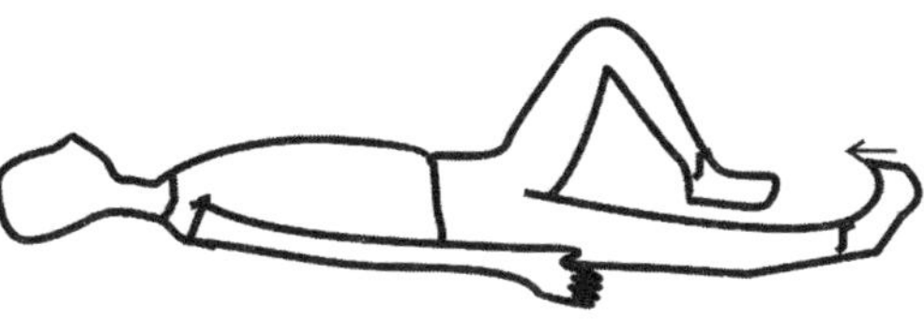

D5.

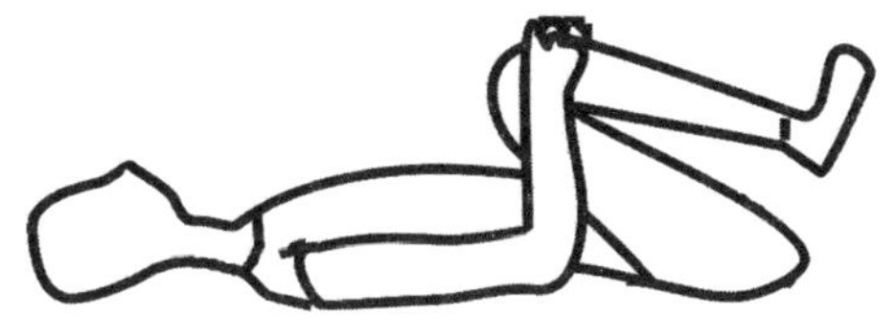

D7.

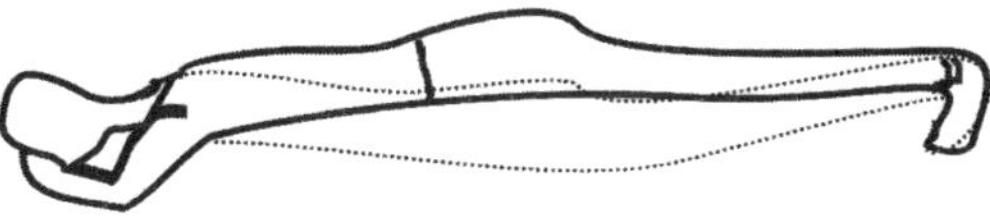

D9.

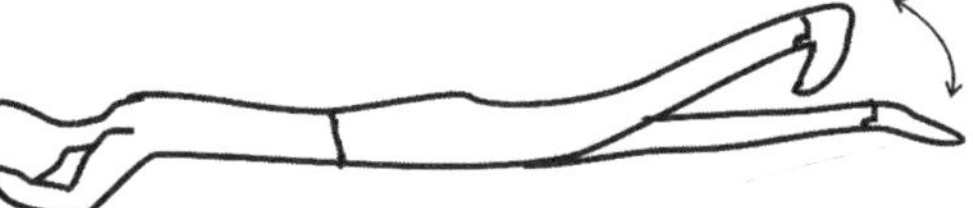

D10.

Sitting

11. Sit on the edge of the chair, with one leg bent, resting on the floor, and the other leg stretched out before you and resting on the heel with your toes pointing towards your head. Lift the straight leg, pushing down at the knee. Switch sides.

12. Sit on a chair with your hands holding the chair and your feet on the ground. Bend your toes so that they are pointing toward your head. Straighten one leg until it is parallel to the ground, stretch the knee, and hold for five seconds. Slowly lower your leg and place it under the chair. Switch sides.

13. Straighten and bend each knee several times before standing.

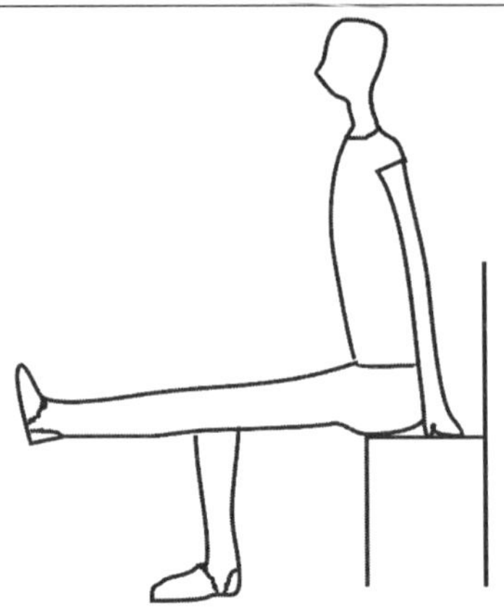

D12.

Standing

The following exercises help energize the body after a long period of sitting, by stimulating the flow of blood and energy toward the feet.

14. Stand with your feet together and arms along your sides. Rise onto the ball of one foot with the other foot flat against the ground. Switch sides (like walking on the spot).

15. Stand with feet apart and hands on your hips. Move your weight from one side of your body to the other. Your knee muscles will contract.

16. With your hands on your hips, slowly stand on tiptoes and go back down again.

17. With your hands on your hips, place one foot forward and move weight forward and back.

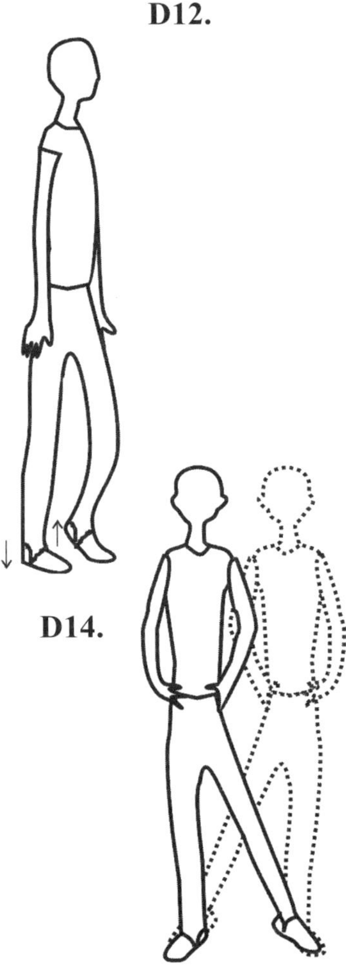

D14.

D15.

174

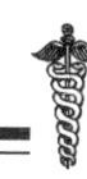

VIII. Case Studies

The states and symptoms that characterize various ailments are analyzed extensively by Eastern medicine. Though this is not the place for in-depth explanations of all the possibilities, I am including several examples of cases from my own practice. By reading the following case studies, you may begin to comprehend and appreciate the differences between the Eastern and Western approaches.

Case #1

H.N.P. is a 37-year-old single male, originally from the United States. He moved to Israel after becoming religiously observant. He currently studies in a Yeshiva (Jewish school) and is boarding with a family. Despite the fact that he is presently moving in Ultra-Orthodox circles, his connection to his family, Israel, and to Judaism is unclear; he still has not "found his place." He wakes up after several hours of sleep, unable to return to his sleep with pains below his navel. He goes to the bathroom frequently and spends a lot of time there. He also suffers from irregularity.

What we have here is a picture of nervous stomach, commonly known as "irritable bowel syndrome." His condition stems from an unsettled lifestyle, poor nutrition, and spiritual and emotional stress. They affect the patient's weak point – his digestive system.

Treatment included lifestyle and nutritional counseling, shiatsu, and acupressure.

Counseling: As part of the treatment plan, we worked towards achieving an organized lifestyle. He was guided regarding how to eat and what to eat. One of the recommendations was to eat light meals comprised of lettuce and oats before bedtime.

Shiatsu and acupressure: The patient learned how to apply repeated, rhythmic pressure to his abdomen from the solar plexus downward, at least three times a day while

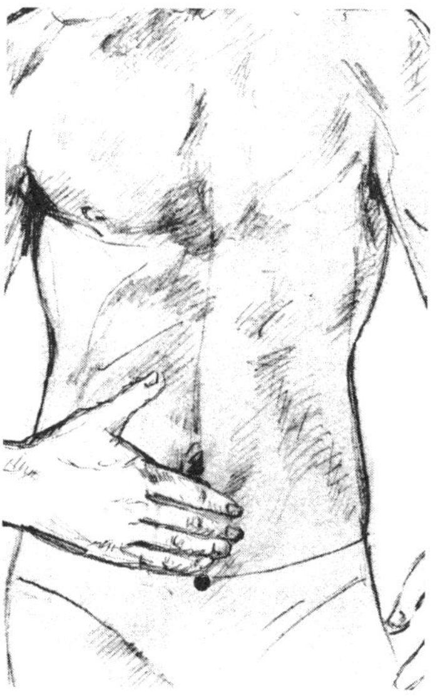

Figure 1

175

inhaling and exhaling. He also learned how to press the following points: CV4 (the width of four fingers below the navel, Figure 1) – for stomach aches and diarrhea, and SP6 (the width of four fingers above the inner ankle, Figure 2) – for insomnia stemming from digestive problems.

After five sessions his stomach attacks were less frequent and less acute, and he also learned how to handle them. At the same time, his sleep became longer and deeper.

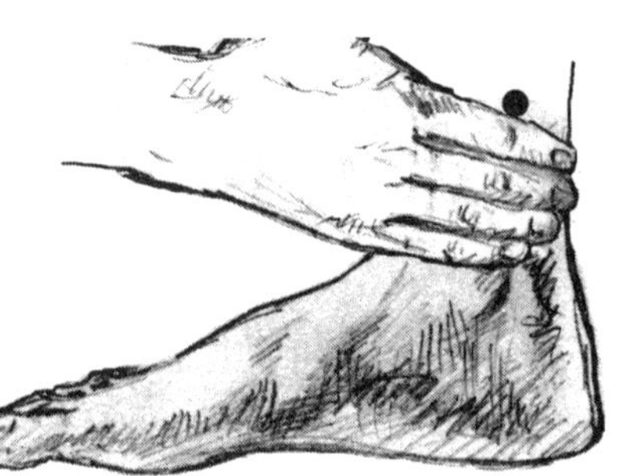

Figure 2

Case #2

According to Chinese medicine, the primary cause of insomnia is a lack of blood, caused by a deficiency or weakness in the heart and spleen. And indeed, the following patient does suffer from a nervous stomach and irregularity, as a result of poor energy flow in the blood, which in turn affected the flow of energy in the body.

A.K. is a single female, aged 25, working as a teacher. A tense personality type to begin with, her stress and fatigue have increased since becoming a teacher. She suffers from insomnia, which manifests in a light sleep from which she wakes easily, difficulty falling asleep, tiredness, and weakness. She is physically "tied up in knots" and is experiencing intestinal problems including irregularity and constipation alternating with diarrhea. She feels a sense of heaviness in and around her eyes and appears pale.

In terms of Chinese medicine, A.K. is suffering from a lack of blood circulation to the heart and spleen with resulting weakness in these organs. Internal damage to the heart and spleen, as well as weakening of the blood, are caused by excessive preoccupation with problems, worry, and fatigue brought on by overwork. The lack of adequate blood supply to the heart impairs its functioning and harms the spirit, resulting in insomnia.

As a first year teacher, the patient is upset by problems in the classroom. She is working very hard to succeed and over-identifying with students' problems. The tension is exhausting her. Her single status, while most of her friends are married with children, also adds to her distress. Stress coupled with too much time spent in contemplation weakens the spleen.

My treatment objective was to strengthen and nourish the heart and

176

spleen to create *chi* and blood, effecting a calming of the spirit for deeper sleep. I used various treatment modes, including shiatsu and acupressure along the meridians of the heart, pericardium, and spleen, to calm and strengthen the heart, relax the body in general, strengthen the spleen and the blood, and regulate the digestive system. Diet to relax and strengthen the body, medicinal herbs for all complaints, and reflexology were suggested. The patient was trained in self-administered reflexology, massage, acupressure, and breathing exercises, and advised to speak with someone to "unload" her troubles.

Reflexology: The self-administered reflexology was based on daily massage for 15 minutes. It included general massage of the feet and special massage of the center of the soles, zones 17–21, and 27–30 (Figure 3).

Massage: This involved massaging the stomach, first clockwise

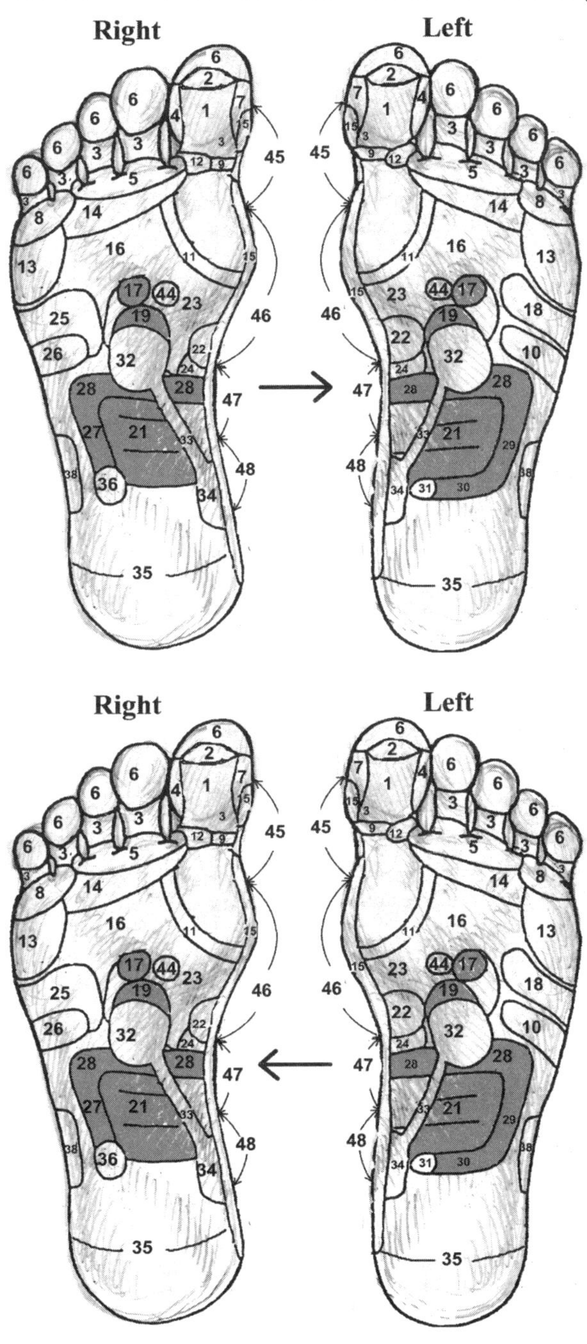

Figure 3

177

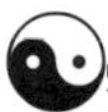

and then counterclockwise (Figure 4).

Acupressure: The patient was trained to press her abdomen, first clockwise and then counterclockwise (Figure 5).

Towards the end of the treatments, A.K. reported that her condition had improved greatly.

Case #3

M.S. is a Yeshiva student, married with three children. Lately, he has been suffering from insomnia, fears, tiredness, and poor concentration. He feels restless and is experiencing heart palpitations and constipation. He also suffers from headaches and neck and back pain. I diagnosed excessive turbulence of the heart and disruption involving the heart and spirit. M.S. recently began learning Kabbalah (Jewish mysticism). He became so deeply involved in its mysteries that he totally lost interest in his regular studies, which frightened him. In addition, his father, a religious court judge, apparently tried to warn him away from over-involvement with Kabbalah.

The fear and intimidation led to anxiety and disruption of the heart and spirit. According to the Chinese perspective, "The spirit did not find a resting place and began to wander." This

178

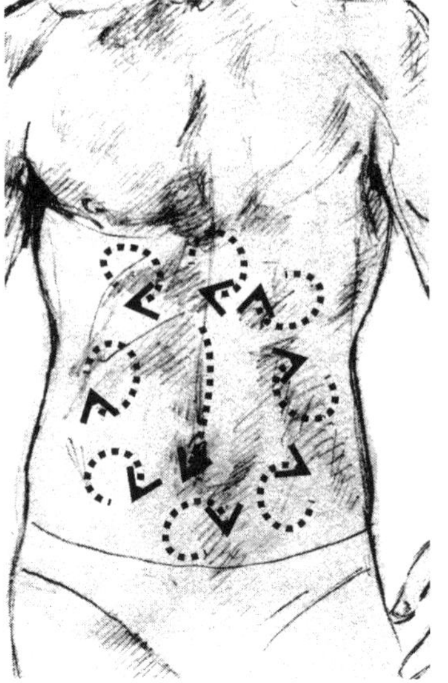

Figure 4

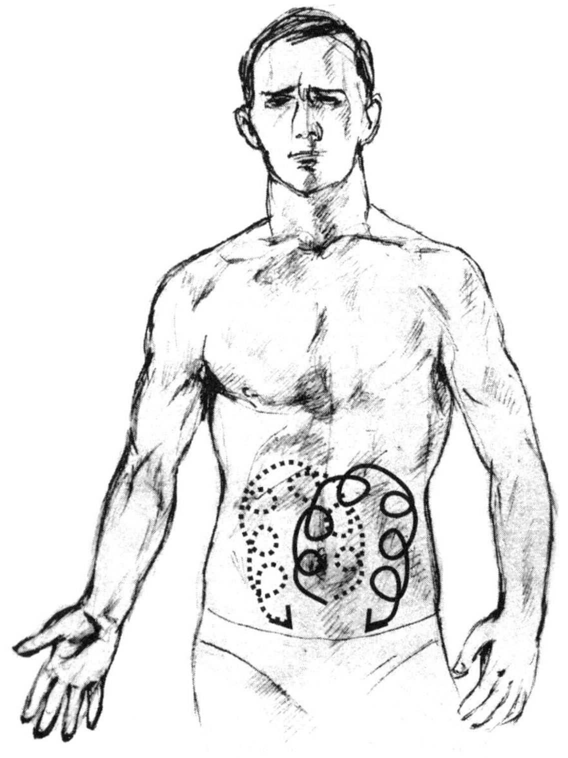

Figure 5

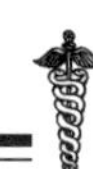

phenomenon was expressed in the patient's symptoms, especially the insomnia. Anxiety, worry, and a busy lifestyle can destroy the *yin* (the body's fluids) due to over-activity of the heart. If this is accompanied by severe emotional problems and anxiety, the result is disrupted sleep and a weakness of the heart.

I suggested that the patient teach part-time, since he liked children, while gradually returning to his studies. In the process of discussing options, including assisting his father-in-law, who ran a school in Europe, it emerged that he felt under pressure to be a "high achiever," which led to his desire for escape. M.S. was advised to take part in physical activity such as bike riding and soccer while slowly building back up to his regular study program.

Treatment included the following techniques, suggestions, and supplements.

Medicinal herbs: In the form of a mixture of Passion Flower, Valeriana, Hops, and Hawthorn (for calming heart palpitations and for strengthening the heart).

Nutritional suggestions: Including plentiful liquids throughout the day andlight foods at night,such as vegetables, especially lettuce, and oatmeal with milk.

Reflexology: The patient received training and guidance in overall massage andgeneral pressure applied to the feet, which represent the entire body. His wife also helped him with reflexology, concentrating on zones 1, 2, 17, and 19 (Figure 6).

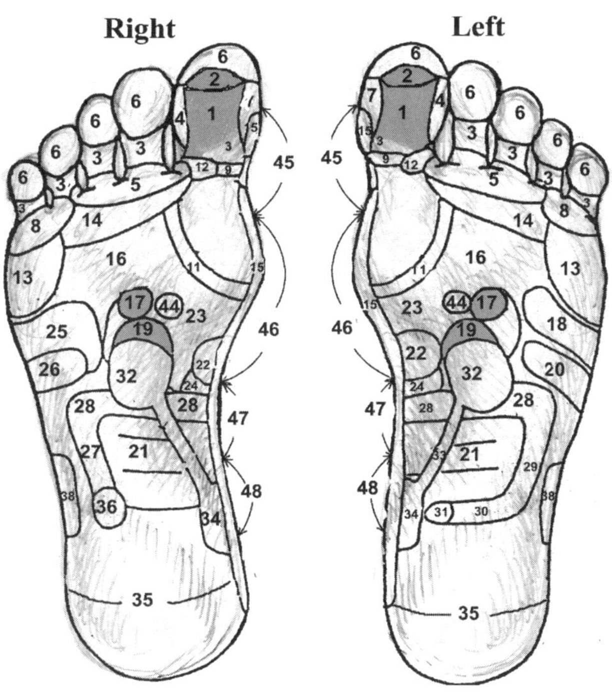

Figure 6

Acupressure: The patient learned to press the following acupressure points as part of his self-administered treatment for insomnia.

Kidney 3 - increases energy of the kidneys and heart (Figure 7)

Heart 7 - calms the heart (Figure 8)

Spleen 6 - the meeting point of three meridians, which calms down over-excitement (Figure 9)

The patient has returned to his regular study program after a period of teaching part time. He reported that after shiatsu treatments he felt much better overall. The fears and anxieties have disappeared and he is taking better care of his health than previously. He feels less pressured and is getting more sleep. He is more relaxed and engages in sports to let off steam. As a result of treatment during the stressful period, the headache and back and neck pain have also disappeared.

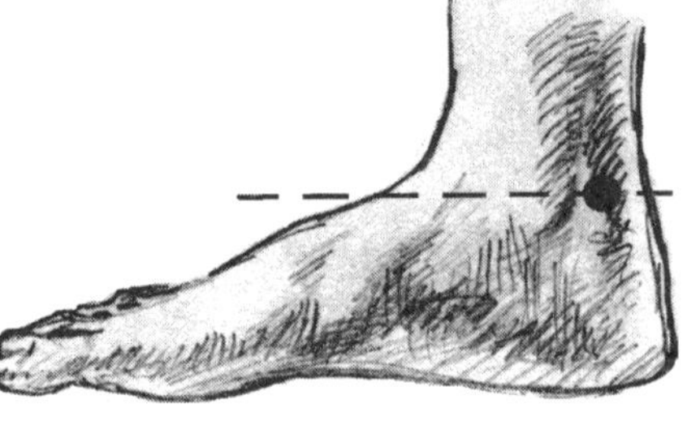

Figure 7

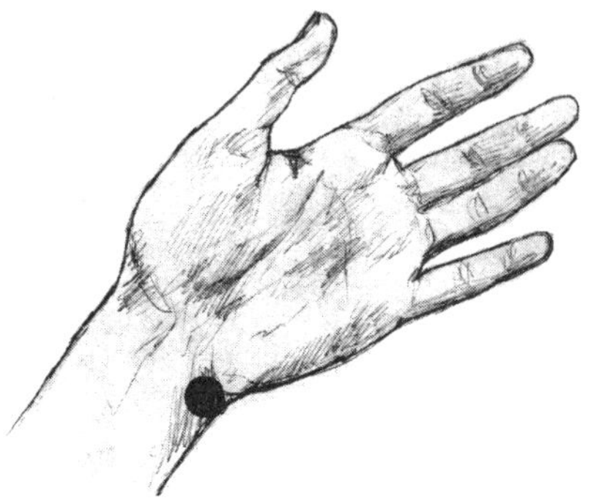

Figure 8

Case #4

E.Y. is a 37-year-old male who works as a clerk in a government ministry. He is the grandson of a well-known political figure. At the start of treatment, he was involved in a relationship with a divorcee and her child from a previous marriage. Later in the treatment process, he married another woman.

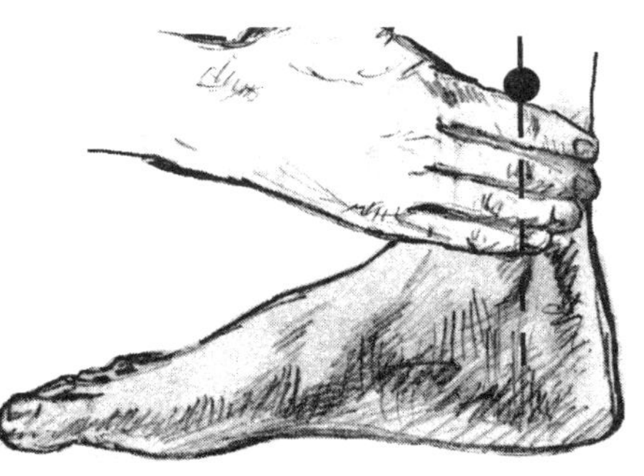

Figure 9

E.Y.'s symptoms included tension, fatigue, skin disorders, allergy, respiratory difficulties, insomnia, frequent colds, a stuffed nose, poor bladder control (he needed to urinate several times during the night), and kidney stones. The breathing difficulties and skin problems had started in childhood. The kidney stones appeared later. His level of stress and anxiety had

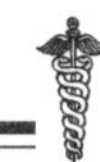

arisen during the period before he sought treatment.

I assessed that his insomnia stemmed from two sources; tension related to his breathing difficulties, and sensitivity of the kidneys, as evidenced by kidney stones and frequent urination. The skin problems are related to the lungs. The feeling of fear is connected to the kidneys and expresses itself as breathing difficulties, which make it hard for him to sleep. His energy is weak, causing the lungs to become blocked because steam is not being brought up to them. The sense of worry is tied to the weak lungs. Frequent colds – apart from the fact that they are associated with the weak lungs and indicate a weakened immune system – point to a weak *jing* (essential energy). This is the underlying reason for his low resistance to illness.

Treatment included the following:

Talk therapy: The patient was encouraged to talk and unload his troubles during the treatment sessions. We analyzed how his girlfriend was manipulating him, and I was able to show him how he was apparently also gaining something from this ambiguous, uncommitted situation. My aim was to strengthen his ability to cope in two areas; breaking off his relationship with this woman and dealing with the pressure from his parents. I also referred the patient to an assertiveness training group.

Reflexology: I focused on the areas of the foot corresponding to the lymphatic system, the adrenal gland, the thymus, the lung region and solar plexus, i.e., zones 16–19 (Figure 10).

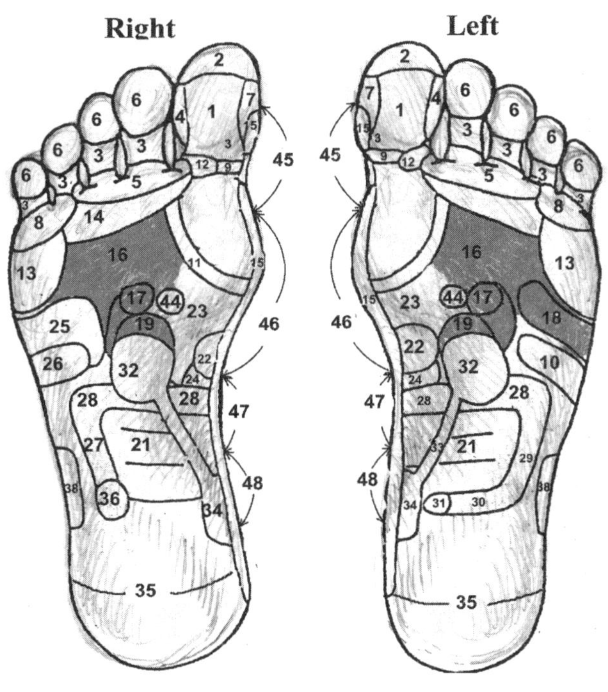

Figure 10

Acupressure: The patient learned to press the following acupressure points:

Kidney 4 - related to the brain; for treatment of mental and emotional problems; effective against fear and anxiety; good for strengthening the essence of the kidneys and the soul or spirit (Figure 11).

Lung 7 - boosts lung functioning, disperses the energy of the air element throughout the body (Figure 12).

Kidney 6 - to strengthen the *yin* (fluids) and sooth the throat (Figure 13).

Pericardium 6 - soothes the soul, calms the heart, and regulates the circulation of the *chi* (energy) (Figure 14).

Dietary changes: Included eliminating dairy products, red meat, and coffee from his diet to reduce stimulating and mucous-producing foods. It was suggested that he eat more unprocessed foods (whole-wheat bread, brown rice, whole grains, etc.), oatmeal for its calming effect, and alfalfa sprouts for increased energy.

Nutritional supplements: Were used to help relax, strengthen, and increase resistance, including foods rich in:

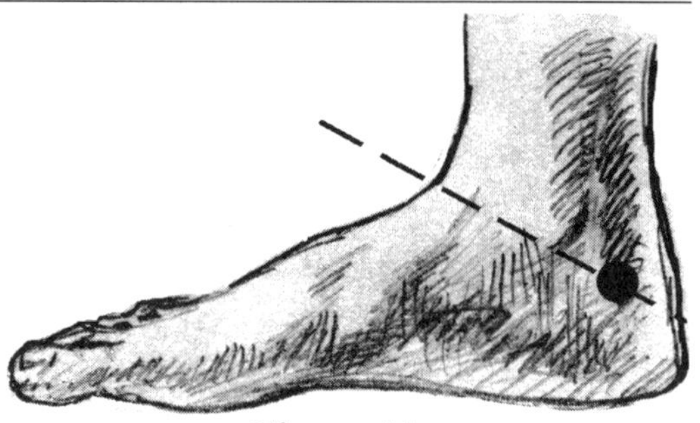

Figure 11

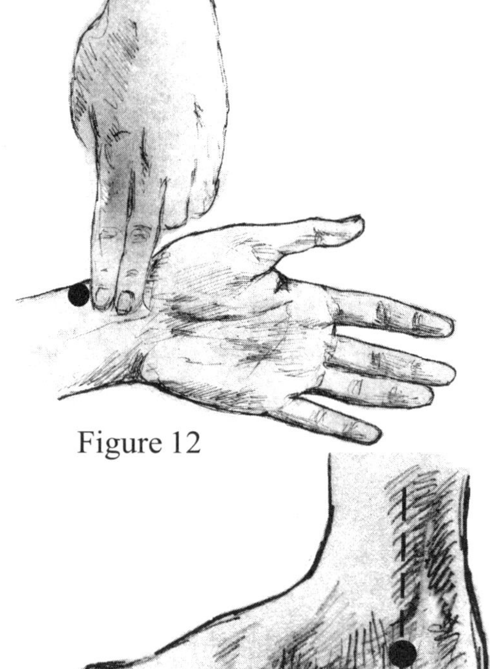

Figure 12

Figure 13

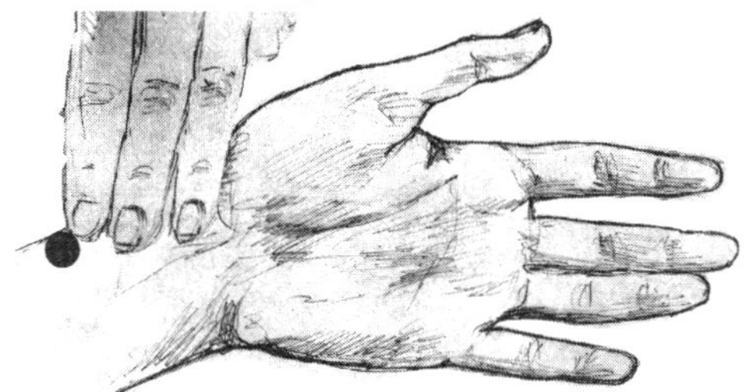

Figure 14

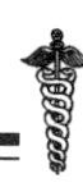

Vitamin C – to reduce fatigue
Vitamin B complex – to relax and strengthen
Vitamin B6 – without yeast, due to suspected allergy
Propolis or Pollen – to increase energy

Medicinal herbs: Echinacea (Cone Flower) and Hydrastis (Golden Seal) were suggested for the immune system. Passion Flower, Melissa (Balm) Hawthorn, and Lavender were suggested for relaxation and sleep.

Shiatsu and Chinese massage: Both were utilized and taught to the patient to treat various organ and system functions and energy flow, including meridians of the heart, lungs, pericardium; the triple warmer, located on the arm; the kidney meridian on the chest; and the lung area by working the conception vessel meridian. (See meridian map, Chapter II).

Exercise: The patient participated in swimming, bike riding, and breathing exercises.

The patient stated that the shiatsu, reflexology, and discussions helped reduce his tension. The self-administered treatments were very helpful in times of stress and tension; they helped him function better on the job and to advance professionally. Following his marriage, his condition improved further, as there were fewer social pressures. The patient's mother said to me, "You've saved my son!"

Case #5

L.P. is a retired male, aged 65. His wife suffers from a degenerative ailment of the muscles, and his son studies in a university. The patient's major complaint is insomnia. Additional problems include an enlarged prostate, frequent need to urinate at night, nervousness, tenseness, heart palpitations, dizziness, fatigue, and migraines. His tension and nervousness escalated with the approach of his retirement and the worsening of his wife's condition. Following retirement, his insomnia intensified. It is difficult for him to fall asleep, and once he does, he only sleeps for two hours. He wakes frequently to urinate and suffers from pain in the knees and back.

According to Chinese medicine, the patient has a deficiency in the *yin* and the *yang* of the kidneys. There is a disharmony, or imbalance, between the heart and the kidneys. The insomnia results from a chronic and damaging deficiency in the fluid of the kidneys, which is then unable to nourish the heart, leading to disharmony between the heart and kidneys, and can lead to high blood pressure.

Frequent waking during the night and the inability to fall asleep again indicates a problem with the heart. Insomnia and fatigue can also result from a reduced level of *chi* (energy) in the heart. As people age, they experience a weakness of the heart and kidneys, which can also be expressed in back pain.

Insomnia-related dizziness is usually associated with the liver. Insufficient blood coupled with overheating of the liver leads to dizziness and insomnia. The condition of his prostate points to a reduction in the *yang* of the kidneys. Finally, a lack of *chi* and blood, along with emotional problems stemming from fear, can result in heart palpitations.

The primary treatment objectives were to calm the heart and soothe the spirit. These involved strengthening of the *yin* and *yang*, thus increasing the amount of fluids in the body; boosting the energy level in general; and calming and reducing the fire of the heart (tension).

Treatment modes included:

Shiatsu: Was applied to several points to reduce heat, boost energy, and promote sleep.

Medicinal herbs: Blossoms of the Sabra fruit (Opuntia) – for prostate.

Echinacea (Cone Flower) and Equisetum (Horse Tail) – for immunization.

Mixture of Hamamelis (Witch Hazel), Plantago (Plantain), and Comfrey in a warm bath – for relaxation.

Oats, Lavender, Verbena, Hops, Nepeta, Passion Flower – for sleep.

Dietary suggestions: Oats, barley, corn, peas, rye, wheat, almonds, beets, cabbage, corn oil, dates, lettuce, mushrooms, peanuts, pistachio nuts, unroasted pumpkin seeds, potato, sweet potato, rice, and soya beans were suggested for nervousness and fatigue.

Nutritional supplements: The patient was advised to eat foods rich in the following:

Vitamin B complex – to strengthen and calm

Vitamin C – to reduce fatigue, also good for the prostate

Exercise: Walking and breathing exercises

Acupressure: The patient learned to press the following acupressure points.

Large intestine 4 – anti-pain point; good also for headaches and insomnia (Figure 15).

Triple warmer 17 – ear point; effective against dizziness, buzzing in the ears, and hearing problems (Figure 16).

Stomach 36 – energy point; used in treating dizziness and knee pain, and in increasing overall energy (Figure 17).

Additional recommendations included avoiding sleep during the day, to be replaced by a stroll followed by a short rest, and finding a part-time occupation that suited him.

The patient did not complete treatment, but after only three sessions he reported a noticeable improvement. He is sleeping four hours straight and going to the bathroom less frequently. He feels more relaxed and has begun looking for part-time employment. His wife's condition still makes him anxious and fearful about the future – "I'm afraid for her, but I've stopped taking out my anger on her." He plans to undergo tests to determine if the palpitations and dizziness are connected to an actual heart ailment, and then to continue treatment. In the meantime, he is continuing his self-administered treatment plan.

Case #6

S.G. is a 52 years old American. He immigrated to Israel approximately 20 years ago and works in educational administration, organizing Talmud Torah (Bible) classes and schools.

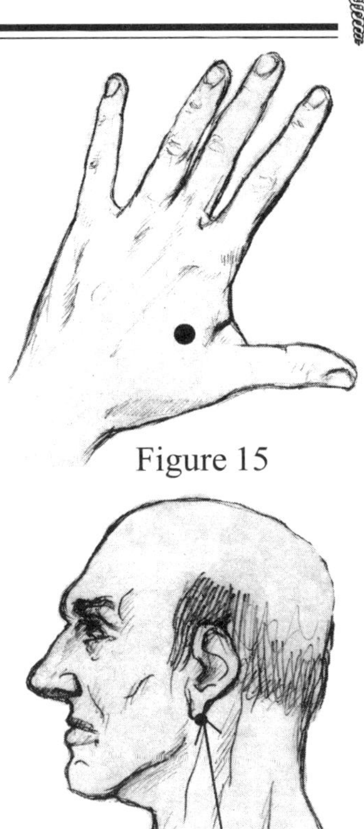

Figure 15

Figure 16

Figure 17

His main symptoms are high blood pressure and diabetes. S.G. is always tense, and suffers from sleep disturbances, cold feet, and sinusitis. 15 years ago he had bronchitis and occasionally suffers from vertigo and impotence. His memory is poor.

S.G. admits that the main cause of his sleep disturbances is stress. Most of his other problems are also stress-related. These problems cause depression and exacerbate the insomnia. For example, headaches caused by hypertension, and cold feet caused by diabetes can lead to insomnia. His wife's frustration with his impotence – caused by diabetes and stress – adds to his stress level, making sleep even more elusive. Thus, the diabetes, impotence, and lack of understanding from his spouse are all factors contributing to his insomnia.

Treatment included counseling, shiatsu, acupressure, and reflexology.

Counseling: We discussed the ways of talking and behaving towards his wife in order to improve their relationship.

Shiatsu: The patient learned to give pressure and massage to his stomach.

Acupressure: He was guided to press any chronic, painful point in his body, especially on his head. (See section about headaches in Chapter III.)

Reflexology: The patient learned to apply general massage to his feet before going to sleep and to sleep with socks.

Today, S.G. functions and sleeps well. His blood pressure has stabilized, his diabetes is under control, and his relationship with his wife has improved as a result of his restored potency. He continues coming for regular preventive treatment and copes well with a busy professional life.

Case #7

K.R. is a married, Polish-born male, and a Holocaust survivor. He is a production technician. Ringing, buzzing, and other sounds in his ears began three years ago, after a serious bout of flu. The ringing in his ears always occurs when he wakes up. After the flu, he became depressed.

K.R. has suffered from migraine headaches for over 30 years. He lived through the Holocaust under extremely harsh conditions and was the only survivor from his family. The migraines began after the war. Recently, he

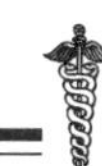

has been suffering from insomnia. He grinds his teeth in his sleep and suffers from receding gums.

In this case, the insomnia is a relatively recent symptom, caused by a build-up of tension, anger, and trauma-induced stress (the Holocaust). Chinese medicine associates tinnitus, migraine, depression, and grinding of the teeth with the emotional (spiritual) part of the liver and gall bladder. Trauma, ill health, and age have depleted the liver and gall bladder, causing a *yin* (body fluids, blood) deficiency in the body and giving rise to insomnia.

The treatment included reflexology, relaxation exercise, acupressure, and herbal medicine.

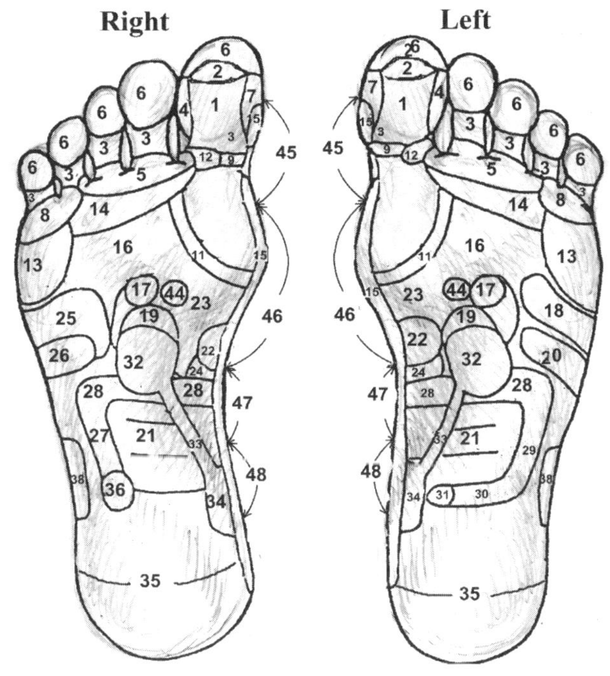

Figure 18

Reflexology: He learned how to apply general massage to his feet, especially the big toe. (Figure 18)

Relaxation exercise: Lying on his bed while keeping his tongue between his teeth and focusing on his mouth area, moving to other bodily sensations in the face and head and focusing on them, too. (See section on tinnitus and migraine in Chapter III.)

K.R. learned to cure his habit of grinding his teeth by doing relaxation exercises. As the attacks of tinnitus and migraine decreased, his insomnia improved.

Herbs: Feverfew was found to be effective in reducing the frequency and severity of the migraines. Hopi auricular candles have prevented further deterioration of his hearing. These candles have an herbal component that cleans out the ear.

After ten treatments, the tinnitus, if it occurs at all, is far less jarring and the migraines are less frequent and less acute. He has learned to administer self-help acupressure as soon as he feels the onset of a migraine or tinnitus. His insomnia has disappeared, though sometimes he wakes up early, which is usual at his age.

Case #8

A.Z. is a 50 year old male suffering from an enlarged prostate, impotence, and fatigue. He suffers from sleep disturbances, stomachaches that cause headaches, and trembles when writing. He experiences a burning sensation when urinating, probably because of the prostate, and is extremely tense, due to impending lay-offs at work.

The insomnia is probably caused by his sense of failure, which is triggered by the impotence, and by his anxiety at work.

The treatment included counseling, acupressure, reflexology, and medicinal herbs.

Acupressure: The wife was taught how to help her husband relax and how to "energize" him through acupressure and Chinese massage (Figures 19, 20, 21). This brought the pair even closer. It was also used during treatment.

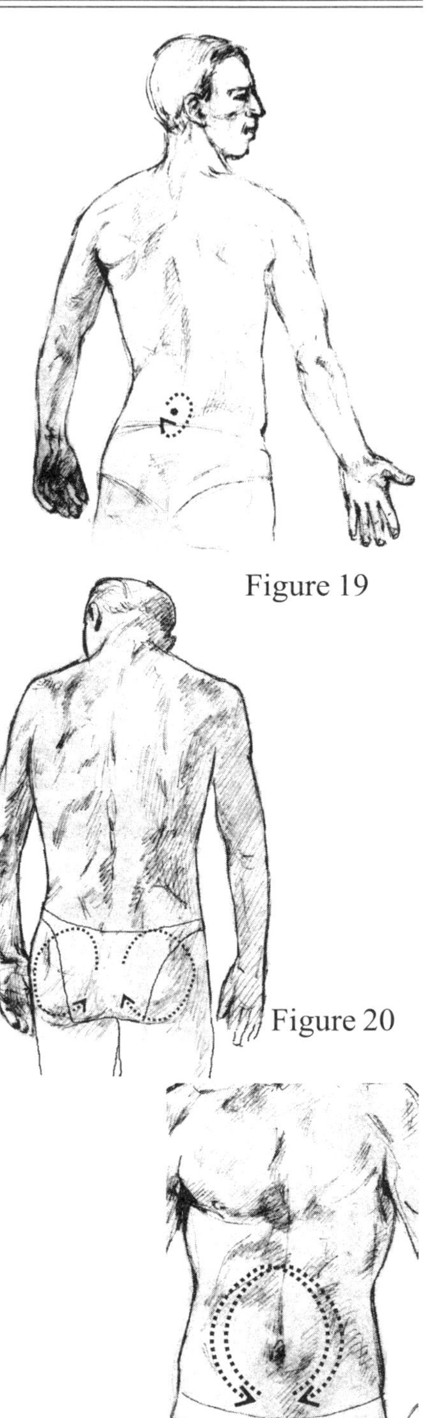

Figure 19

Figure 20

Figure 21

188

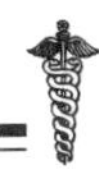

Counseling: Because impotence is a problem that includes the wife, she was also asked to come. She made light of her husband's impotence, saying the problem was not as bad as he made it out to be, and was not causing her particular hardship. She did not value her husband any less because of it. Nor did she think less of him because of the threatened lay-off, which according to her was caused by the company's financial problems, rather than by her husband's performance at work. This assurance, given by the wife in the therapist's presence calmed the patient and "validated" him.

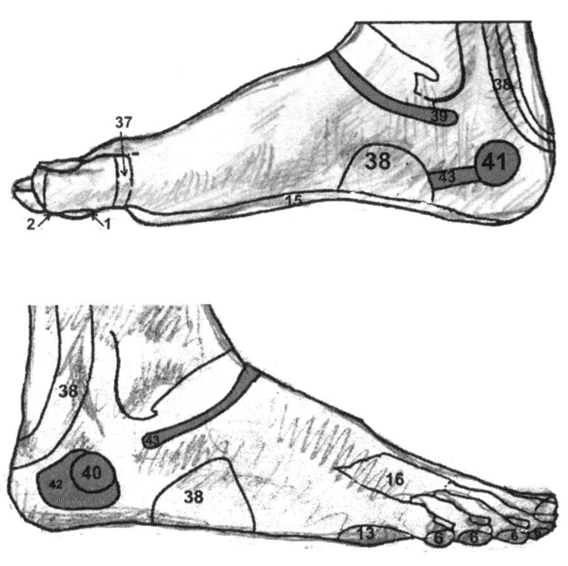

Figure 22

Reflexology: The wife learned to apply general massage to his feet, especially to zones 39 - 43. (Figure 22).

Herbs: He was also given potency-enhancing herbs (Ginseng) and prostate reducing herbs (Cacti).

His enlarged prostate has improved, and he no longer needs surgery. His physical relationship with his wife has improved and he was not laid off, partly because he has learned to become more assertive and to fight for his job. When A.Z. finished treatment, after ten sessions, he was in high spirits.

Children's Cases

Case study 1: A.B.

A.B. is seven years old. He began wetting his bed two years ago, right after the birth of his younger brother. Along with this brother, he has two younger sisters and four older siblings. There are eight children in the family, ranging in age from two to twelve. A.B. is a "sandwich" child.

The mother is a housewife and teacher, while the father studies full time at a Yeshiva

The mother can barely cope. The oldest child, a girl aged 12, helps the mother look after the other children and often stays at home when the mother can't find a babysitter. The father is busy studying. The only available time he has to help at home is in the mornings, between 8-9. In the afternoon, he takes a siesta before returning to the Yeshiva. He gets back late in the evening. Even on Shabbat he is busy, although it's the only day he has a little time for the children.

The underlying cause: The boy himself pointed to the main cause of the problem, namely lack of attention. Even on Shabbat, his father studies with all the children, not with him alone. Sometimes, when the father goes to the synagogue, he leaves A.B. behind. When I inquired as to the immediate cause of the bedwetting, the mother replied that he is jealous of his siblings, although the birth of his younger sisters did not affect him as much as that of his younger brother. He often does not want to go to school), and pretends he is ill in order to stay at home. At first the parents tried to take no notice of his bedwetting problem – but now, they are at their wits' end.

When I asked why they took no notice of the problem, they replied that they thought the problem was probably genetic. The boy's uncles and even his siblings had bedwetted until late. They pointed out that their son had, to their great delight, become dry at an early age, before he began bedwetting again.

Treatment: Treatment consisted of: (a) counseling the parents and child, (b) reflexology, (c) diet and dietary supplements, (d) herbal medicines, (e) shiatsu, and (f) Chinese massage.

(a) *Counseling*: We discussed with the parents the causes of the prob-

190

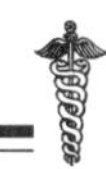

lem, and how to deal with it. We suggested they praise and encourage the child, and give him positive reinforcement through prizes, both during the intermediate and final stages of his treatment. We discussed the possibility of accompanying the child to the toilet before he went to bed, and possible reaction to this. In our talks with A.B. we tried to offer him the opportunity of venting his feeling. In the course of our conversation, he said that at home he often felt "as if he simply weren't there." His mother was busy all the time with the housework, and any spare time she had was devoted to preparing lessons and marking tests. As to his father, "he just never got to speak to him."

In a joint session with A.B. and his parents, we raised these points. We decided to try and improve the relationship between father and child. We arranged for the father to learn with the child individually, particularly on the Shabbat but also for a short while each afternoon. Likewise, we agreed that the boy would visit the father occasionally at the Yeshiva, and come home with him in the evening. A.B. requested that his father take him to the toilet each night (he was not willing for his mother to take him). In a session together with his older siblings, A.B. was able to tell them that it upset him that they made fun of him.

(b)*Reflexology*:We taught the father how to give a general massage to the soles of his son's feet (Figure 1).

(c) *Diet and dietary supplements*: We recommended a reduction in sugar intake and an increase in fruits and vegetables, especially those rich in vitamin C, to strengthen the system.

(d) *Herbal medicines*: We recommended

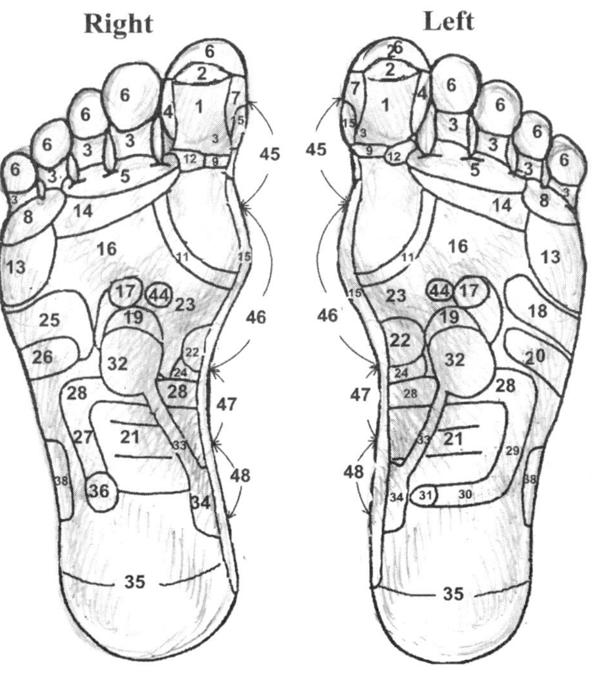

Figure 1

Passiflora (Passion Flower), Echinacea (Cone Flower), Urtica (Nettles) and Alfalfa (Lucerne).

(e) *Acupressure*: We taught the father to apply pressure at the following points:
- ◆ neck point (Figure 2)
- ◆ foot point (Figure 3)
- ◆ lower stomach point (Figure 4)
- ◆ ankle point (Figure 5)

(f) *Chinese massage*: We taught the father to apply the following massages:
- ◆ Supporting the spine (Figure 6)
- ◆ Opening the gate of life (Figure 7)
- ◆ Brushing down (Figure 8 - page 194)

The father applied these treatments (reflexology, acupressure,

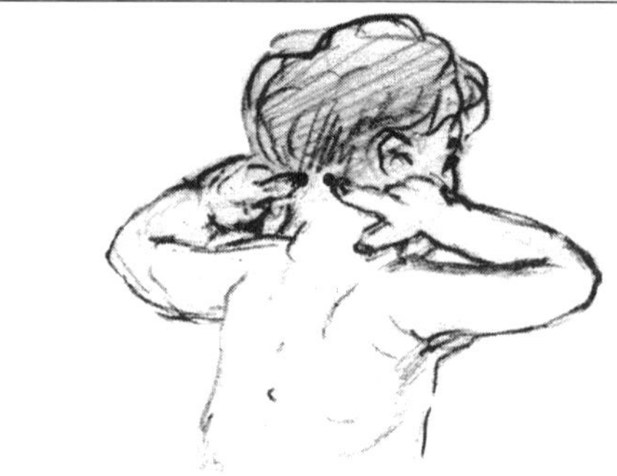

Figure 2

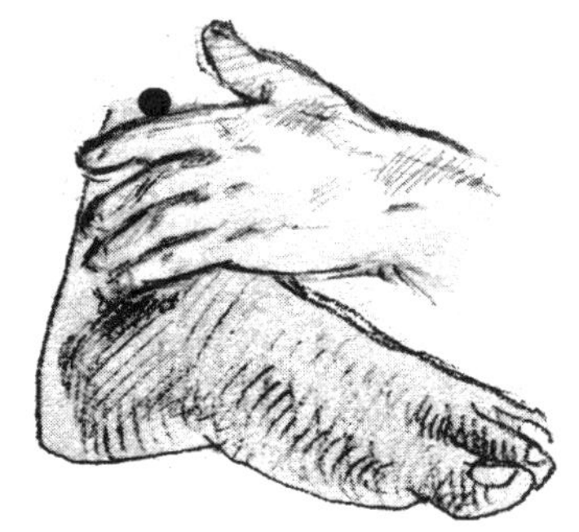

Figure 3

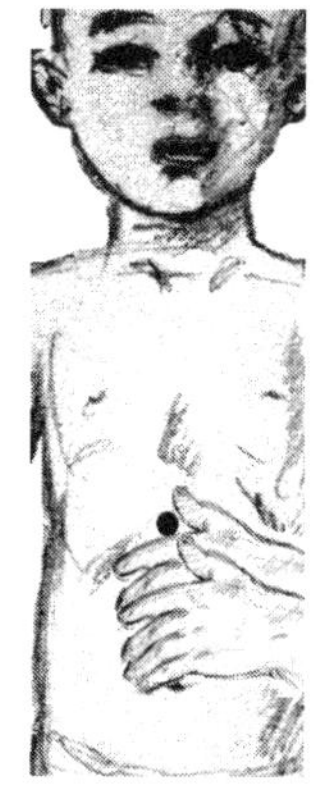

Figure 4

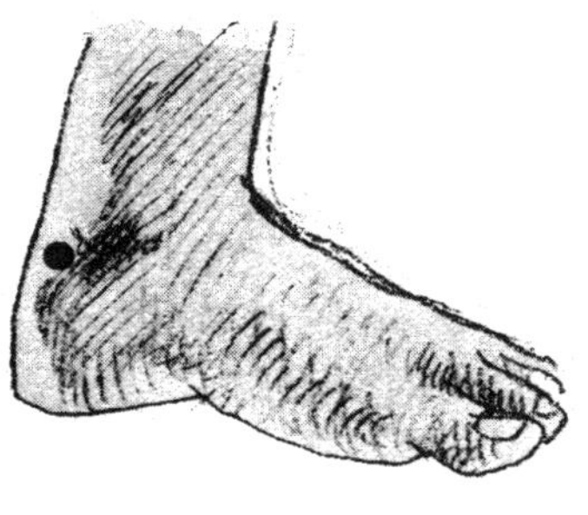

Figure 5

and the Chinese massage) alternately. Later, the child learnt to do acupressure on himself. The parents cooperated with us, and tried hard to solve the problem. Their efforts paid off. After five treatments, there was a marked improvement, and after ten treatments, the child remained dry.

A.B. himself summarized his cure by saying: "Now I have a friend." When asked who his friend was, he smiled, pointed to his father and said: "My father."

Case study 2: B.G.

B.G. is five years old, and has two older brothers aged 11 and 13. Her parents are middle aged (around 50).

As a baby, B.G. suffered form spastic bronchitis, and since age two, has been suffering from chronic colds. She constantly has a runny nose, and is always catching colds. Frequently, these colds are accompanied by an excruciating earache.

Usually the colds begin with a sore throat which gets progressively worse. B.G. typically develops a high fever which lasts about a week. The colds occur in the summer, too.

The mother is of the school that believes "children must develop their own resistance." This approach has worked with her two older children, and she cannot understand why it does not work with her daughter.

The girl's father is very hard to get hold of (I tried, in vain, to get hold of him). He is a businessman who is often abroad and even when he is in the country, he leaves the children's education up to the mother.

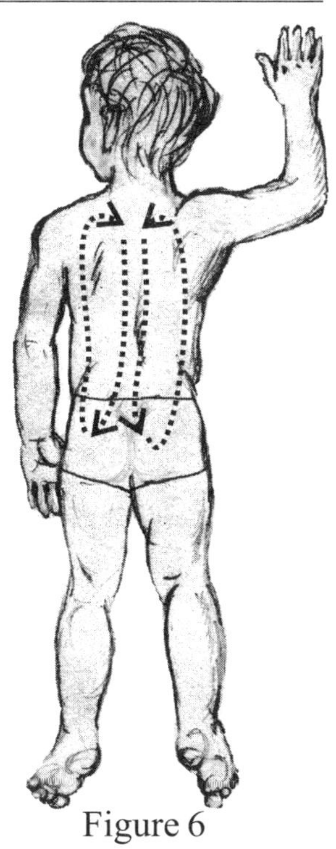

Figure 6

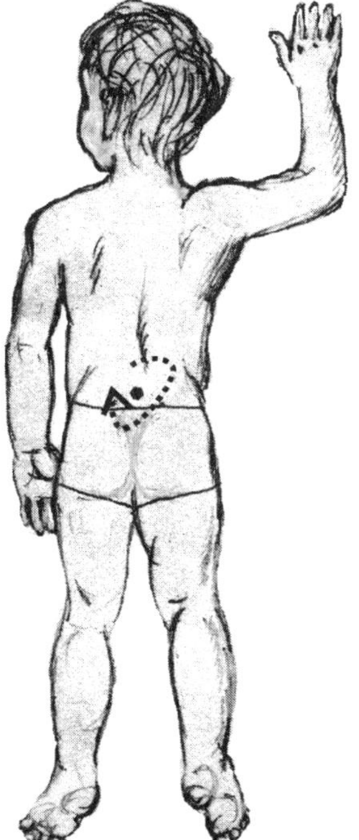

Figure 7

Treatment: Treatment consisted of: (a) counseling the mother, (b)herbal medicines, (c) acupressure, (d) diet and supplements.

(a) *Counseling the mother*: Initially, the mother, who is very self-assured and opinionated, was resistant to counseling, but at her husband's urgings, she agreed to go. During sessions, she discovered that underneath her strong front, she was actually not as strong as she seemed, and even wondered if her approach was right. She felt she simply "couldn't carry on." She began to realize that she had been too strict toward her daughter.

Once she began accepting her daughter for who she was, she was able to cooperate with the treatment. She learned how to bring down the child's fever when it was high, and to encourage the girl to drink, rather than eat when she was unwell. She also learned how to treat other symptoms of chronic flu and colds, such as acute earaches (with warm salt in a cloth bag over the ear, see section on Children's Colds Chapter IV).

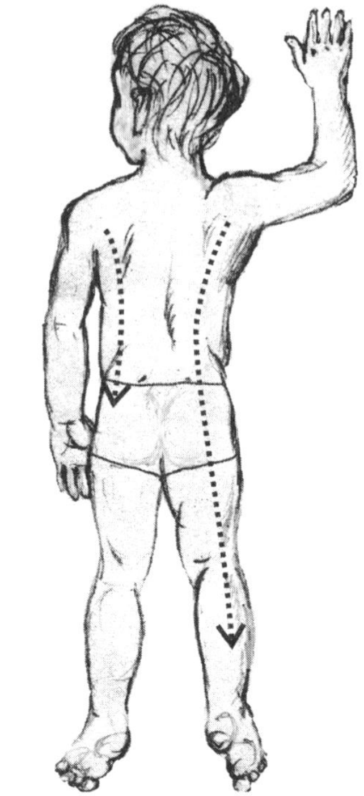

Figure 8

(b) *Herbal medicines*: The following were recommended for strengthening the immune system:

Echinacea (Cone Flower)
Equisetum (Horsetail)
Alfalfa (Lucerne)
Achillea (Yarrow)
Taraxacum (Dandelion).

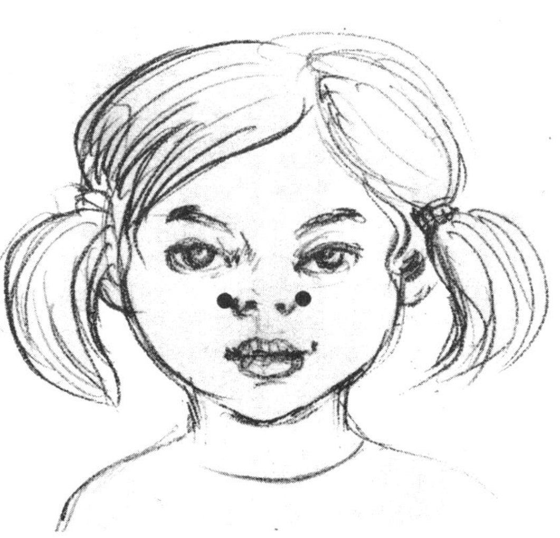

Figure 9

194

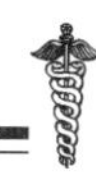

(c) *Acupressure*: We taught the mother the following acupressure points:

1. For a runny or blocked nose: points around the nose (Figure 9).

2. For aches and pains in general and sore throat in particular, points on the flat of the hand that eliminate pain (Figure10).

3. For coughs and colds in general, a lung point situated nears the wrist (Figure 11). (See section about Children's Colds Chapter IV).

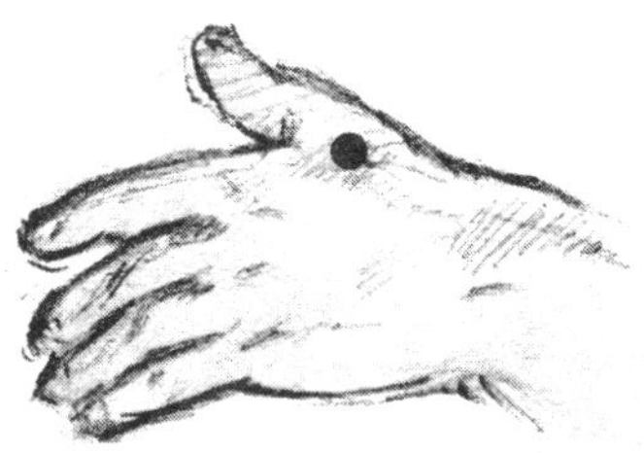

Figure 10

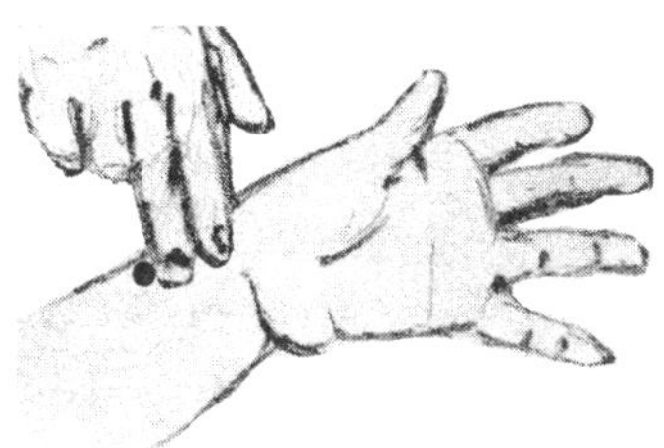

Figure 11

(d) *Diet*: The mother changed the girl's diet to include plenty of fruit and vegetables (especially those rich in vitamin C, such as broccoli, guava, red peppers, melon, citrus fruit, kiwi, strawberries, etc.) and whole grains. Likewise, she reduced her intake of foods containing refined flour, white sugar, etc.

After about five treatments over a period of two weeks, the girl's situation improved, and she was free of colds for the following two weeks.

The mother continued treating the child, and a month later phoned me to tell me that although the girl had caught a cold, it was less severe than usual and had lasted only three days.

Today the girl suffers less from a runny nose, coughs only infrequently, and is altogether in better shape.

195

IX. Conclusion

With this book, I have attempted to demonstrate how to apply an all-encompassing, holistic approach to the treatment of persons suffering from various ailments. In addition, I have analyzed both the Western and Eastern viewpoints regarding both the underlying causes of ailments and the ways in which various ailments can be treated.

The ostensible clash between the two approaches is, however, mostly one of methodology. In the first place, this is because both outlooks have drawn steadily closer to a common ground in recent decades, even becoming somewhat integrated. In the aftermath of World War II – with increased contact between the West and the East and the lowering of the Bamboo Curtain – the West waxed enthusiastic about the wisdom of Chinese medicine, while the encounter between Eastern and Western culture generated Eastern enthusiasm for sophisticated Western medicine. Thus my intention has been to propose a possible merger between the two approaches – a low-key and moderate integration riding the wave of the two approaches' instantaneous connection.

Secondly, even when enumerating Western methods of treatment, I have focused on more holistic, natural, complementary approaches and less on conventional ones. It is therefore not surprising that medicinal herbs, aromatherapy and especially reflexology have been included in this category.

As for the ailments themselves, I have attempted first and foremost, to demonstrate that they are to be viewed as individual, subjective problems – an attitude typical of the Eastern approach to medicine. When a person is satisfied with his or her level of health and functioning, this is an acceptable state of affairs. The problem arises when he or she is not satisfied, in all senses of the word. It is then that we are called on to step in. This does not mean to say that we should immediately descend upon the patient with the full range of techniques, approaches and herbs in our arsenal, but rather that we should select what is appropriate for that particular patient – in the opinion of both the patient and the healer. It is entirely conceivable that we will choose only one method of tackling the problem, but even in such a case, it must be an all-encompassing, holistic approach. Why is this so? Because we are relating to the person as a whole. As it is written in *The Ethics of The Fathers*, "One should welcome the whole person with warmth."

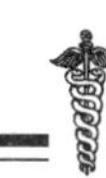

To highlight this concept, I have presented case histories of patients, each of whom I treated with a different method in accordance with his or her specific needs and my personal skills and experience. (As an interesting side note, a young male made the comment to me that perhaps the reason why shiatsu had helped him so much was because it involved greater physical contact and personal interaction than acupuncture.)

In natural medicine, we view the patient not only as a lone individual but also in conjunction with his or her environment; thus, in helping the patient, we are also helping those around him or her who are "suffering" in their own way due to the patient's problem. Consequently, when a mother says, "You've succeeded in saving my son," I take this to mean that I have aided her as well.

Above all, throughout the book, I have attempted to present the Jewish viewpoint in regard to natural healing. In fact, there are some who see the origins of Eastern wisdom, and thus Chinese medicine, in Judaism.

> *Abraham willed all that he owned Isaac; but to Abraham's sons by concubines Abraham gave gifts while he was still living, and he sent them away from his son Isaac eastward, to the land of the East.* Genesis 25.5-6

What is the meaning of "gifts"? Not silver or gold, since Abraham had already given everything to Isaac, but gifts of wisdom. The commentators say he taught them "to banish the demons." Here we have a source for one of the traditional ways of healing.

There is also a tradition that some of the Ten Tribes were exiled to China. There are indications that at that period in time, a change occurred in Chinese philosophy, which made it more in keeping with the outlook of Judaism.

Chinese medicine is strongly anchored in the philosophical outlook of the days of Confucianism and Taoism. It seems to me that Confucianism is the philosophic school that comes closest to Judaism; claiming that a man must meet his forefathers (when he passes from this world) in a state of wholeness. This is similar to a concept in Judaism. As a result of this perspective, acupuncture, herbal remedies and other relatively non-invasive techniques are preferable to surgery or invasive techniques.

X. About the Author

Yehonatan Sraya was born in Jerusalem, in 1935, to parents from Yemen. His first "hands-on" experience in performing acupressure was as a young child under his grandmother's tutelage.

Dr. Sraya has a B.A. in special education and an M.A. in educational and psychological counseling from The Hebrew University. He has spent many years teaching and counseling in the field of education. He first studied acupressure in England. Subsequently, he became a qualified acupuncturist after four years of studies in Chinese medicine at a branch of the California College of Acupuncture, USA.

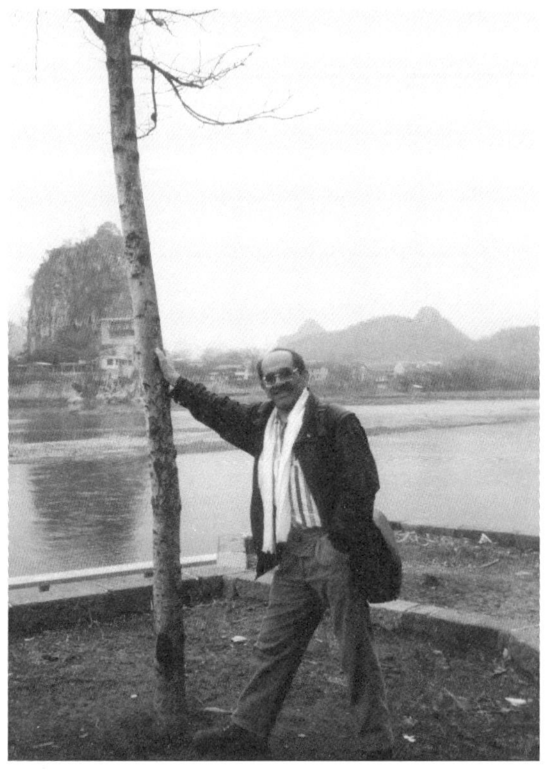

Dr. Sraya received his Ph.D. in Chinese medicine from Newport University, USA, in 1993. Shortly thereafter he led a professional tour to China where he carried out a medical project on sleep disturbances. He then received a certificate of appreciation from the University of Beijing.

For the past decade, Dr. Sraya has been studying Torah intensively. After successfully completing the examinations for Rabbinical ordination, he received Smichat Chachomim in October 1999. Dr. Sraya combines his Torah knowledge and the wisdom of the Rambam with his understanding of Chinese medicine.

Dr. Sraya taught shiatsu at The Popular University and The Hebrew University. He is a popular lecturer who frequently speaks about comprehensive medicine. His articles on "healthy living" have been published in various Israeli periodicals.

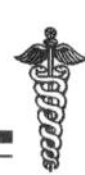

XI. Bibliography

Beijing College
Essentials of Chinese Acupuncture
Foreign Languages Press, China 1980

Berman, D.A.
Pain Relief and Acupuncture
American Journal of Acupuncture, Vol. 7, No. 1, March 1979

Berman, Ya'acov
Nutrition
Privately published, Israel 1983

Carasso, R.
Alternatives in Healing
Marshall Edition Ltd. 1988

Cheung, C.S.
Mental Dysfunction
Traditional Chinese Medical Publisher
San Francisco 1981

Hel-Or, Yom-Tov
Ripui Vitali Tiv'i
Barmatz Publishing, Jerusalem, 1979

Horowitz, Ilan
A Guide for the Practitioner
Hemed Publishing, Jerusalem, 1994

Kaptchuk, J. Ted, O.M.D
The Web that has no Weaver
Congdon and Weed Inc., New York 1983

Levin, Yitzchak
  The World of Sleep and Dreams
  Maariv, Tel Aviv 1981

Mastsumoto, Kiiko and Birch, Stephen
  Five Elements and Ten Stems
  Paradigm Publications, Brookline 1983

Namikoshi, Tokogiro
  Japanese Finger Pressure Therapy
  Japan Publications Inc., Tokyo 1977–1982

O'Connor, John and Benski, Dan
  Acupuncture
  East Land Press, Seattle 1981

Ohashi, Wataru
  Do It Yourself - Shiatsu
  Unwin Paperbacks, London 1977–1985

Olshevsky, Moshe
  The Manual of Natural Therapy
  Facts on File, New York, Oxford 1989

Russell, Stephen and Gordon Yehudi
  Massage for Life
  Gaia Books, London 1985

Scott, J.
  Acupuncture: The Diagnosis and Treatment of Headaches
  Journal of Chinese Medicine 15, May 1984

Shao, L.K.
  Insomnia
  American College of Chinese Medicine No. 15, May 1984